THE GP CONSULTATION
A Registrar's Guide

For

Tessa, Paul and Christopher

In
Memory
of
Keith

Acknowledgements
for the First Edition

I should like to take this opportunity to thank those who have helped and influenced me to write this book. My first real introduction to general practice was as a trainee in Gloucester. Jeremy Barnes, my trainer showed me, by example, the value of obtaining a clear history, undistorted by unnecessary interruptions and, thereby, of allowing the patient greater freedom to express himself in an unhurried way. I should, therefore, like to acknowledge his influence in initiating my special interest in the general practice consultation.

Since then, through countless casual conversations with many general practitioners I have learned to appreciate the different advantages of the varied ways in which we all consult. Clearly it would not be practical to mention all by name, but I would like to include a few who have had a greater influence upon me, my partners John Andrewes, Henry Byrom, and Madeleine Richardson, and my friends Chris Woodyatt of Hull, Roger Unwin of Canterbury, John Quarrie of Maidstone and my brother and his wife, Roger and Oonagh Livesey of Nottingham. All have taught me so much about the undocumented aspects of general practice.

While writing this book, my former partner and friend, Keith Haynes became seriously ill and died at the young age of 44 years. I should like to express a special debt of gratitude to him. Despite considerable ill health and the anguish of knowing he had a relatively short life ahead of him, he remained always an excellent and exemplary general practitioner. Always kind and cheerful, knowledgeable and conscientious he knew what it was like to suffer ill health, and was able to sympathize fully with patients, many of whom were less ill than himself. Together with his sense of humour and gentle, teasing manner he was an ideal partner and a much loved doctor.

For one of the main themes in this book I should like to acknowledge the influence of David Tuckett, whom I met at a trainers course in Cambridge in 1983, and who convinced me of the enormous importance of exploring the patient's own ideas and concerns. For another theme, namely that of marrying the consultation to the patient's and doctor's personalities, I should like to express my gratitude to Professor Veikko Tähkä of Finland.

For their help in correcting the manuscript and for suggesting modifications I am grateful to my trainees, Vanessa Potter and Julie Fegent, both of whom have also taught me much about consulting with patients.

I should also like to take this opportunity to thank Arnold Bloom, medical editor and chairman of the British Diabetic Association who, despite an extremely busy life, took considerable pains to read the manuscript thoroughly and make several valuable suggestions.

In another context, but certainly no less important, I should like to acknowledge the influence of the many co-workers with whom I am in daily contact—nurses, health visitors and receptionists—all of whom have a greater influence upon me than they probably imagine.

In living in Canterbury I have been most fortunate in having free access to the Postgraduate Medical Centre Library, whose librarian, Sue Cover offers a splendid service. I would like to express my gratitude to her for providing most of the reference material with remarkable and friendly efficiency and for laboriously typing the text from my original manuscript. I should also like to acknowledge her helpful comments.

My thanks are also due to the following for permission to reproduce extracts from copyright materials:

Adam Hilger, Bristol: *Mould's Medical Anecdotes* (1984), by Richard Mould.

Adis: Health Science Press, Sydney: *The Patient–Doctor Relationship* (1984), by Veikko Tähkä.

British Medical Association Planning Unit Report 1970: *Report of the Working Party on Primary Medical Care.*

Chapman & Hall, London and Penguin Books Ltd, Harmondsworth: *Brideshead Revisited* (1945), by Evelyn Waugh. Reprinted by permission of A. D. Peters & Co. Ltd.

Geoffrey Bles, London: *Will Pickles of Wensleydale; Life of a Country Doctor* (1970), by John Pemberton.

HMSO, London: (republished by Royal College of General Practitioners) *Doctors Talking to Patients* (1976), by P. S. Byrne and B. E. L. Long.

HMSO, London: *The Doctor–Patient Relationship* (1979), by F. Fitton and H. W. K. Acheson.

The Hogarth Press, London and Penguin Books Ltd, Harmondsworth: *The Seed and the Sower* (1963), by Sir Laurens van der Post.

Hogarth Press, London: *This Island Now* (1963), by G. M. Carstairs.

John Wright, Bristol: *Epidemiology in Country Practice*, by W. N. Pickles. Published in 1939 and reissued in 1949.

E. S. Livingstone Ltd, Edinburgh and London: *Clinical Examination* (1967), edited by J. Macleod.

Oxford Medical Publications: *The Consultation: An Approach to Learning and Teaching* (1984), by D. Pendleton *et al.*

Oxford University Press, Nuffield Provincial Hospitals Trust: *Good General Practice* (1954), by Lord Taylor.

Pitman Medical, London: *The Doctor, his Patient and the Illness* (1964), by M. Balint.

Regional Doctor Publication Ltd, London: Foreword to *Patient Centred Medicine* (1972), by Professor Lord Rosenheim.

Routledge and Kegan Paul, London and Boston: *Going to See the Doctor* (1975), by G. Stimson and B. Webb.

Weidenfeld and Nicholson, London: *Doctors* (1984), by Jonathan Gathorne-Hardy.

Finally, I am indebted to my wife, to a greater degree than she will allow me to express here, for her support and help with correcting the manuscript.

Though acknowledging the help and influence of all concerned I would like to accept full responsibility for all the opinions expressed and any subsequent errors that may come to light in the future.

Chapter 1

Introduction

*'If [a doctor] can give time to listen with sympathy, he can probably
do more than a cataract of medicine to cleanse the stuffed bosom of
that perilous stuff that weighs upon the heart.'*
John Pemberton—*Will Pickles of Wensleydale*

Dr Pickles of Wensleydale frequently introduced his lectures on general
practice with this marvellously graphic description.

'I recall a particularly lovely evening in early summer, when I
climbed alone to the summit of one of our noble hills. The sun was
setting and it lit up the grim pile of an ancient castle, once the
prison of history's unhappiest queen, our little lake seemed to lie at
my feet and one by one I made out most of our grey villages with
their thin pall of smoke. And as I watched the evening train
creeping up the valley with its pauses at our three stations, a quaint
thought came into my head and it was that there was hardly a man,
woman, or child in all those villages of whom I did not know the
Christian name and with whom I was not on terms of intimate
friendship.'

Such an idealized view makes no mention of the frustration and exasperation which is the lot of all general practitioners. Yet for all its in-
completeness, it embodies an aspiration that I suspect most general
practitioners hold at some time, and suggests a relationship with the
doctor that most patients would welcome. If this is the frequent aim of
most doctors and the hope of most patients, why does the relationship
between patient and doctor frequently go sour?

Surveys between 1964 and 1981 by Ann Cartwright confirm that
contact with people and the feelings that prevail between them have
remained the main sources of satisfaction for most doctors, while the
most important attributes that patients feel their doctors should possess
are friendliness and a caring manner. These are, of course, not the only
requirements for a successful relationship between doctor and patient.
Nevertheless, if they are important aspirations, it is paradoxical that our
aims seem to contrast widely with our practice. In 1976 Byrne and Long
(recently republished by the RCGP in 1984) transcribed audiotaped
interviews of real consultations and analysed the findings. It seemed that
the aim of most doctors they investigated was to usher the patient out of

the surgery as quickly and efficiently as possible, a conclusion which is at once both regrettable and amusing.

No doubt it reflects the ambivalence of the doctor–patient relationship, the reality rather than the ideal, and must indicate some of the irritation that all doctors feel for their patients from time to time. Many books have been written which attempt to teach the medical student how to take a case history and how to examine a patient. For various reasons this hospital-based technique is not easily applicable to general practice. Most general practitioners have, by trial and error, modified the techniques they were taught in medical school, and to the trainee GP observer such abbreviated methods must seem impulsive, perhaps intuitive or even foolhardy. The main aim of this book, therefore, is to explain to the trainee what the general practitioner is seeking to achieve, and how to make sense of the brief consultations that he may witness during the course of his training. It has also been my purpose to suggest ways in which improvements in the GP consultation may be made and to give some direction for the trainee to follow. In attempting this I hope to suggest only that which is practicable, reasonable and sensible.

General Practitioners and Specialists

Are general practitioners practising medicine in a different way from hospital colleagues? Or are we striving to perform the same role with less knowledge and poorer facilities? There are some GPs who would like to consider themselves as specialists in their own field, but I suspect most of us feel unattracted by this spurious concept. It does seem obvious that we are not the same as our hospital colleagues; we have different objectives, form a different relationship with our patients, have a greater knowledge about individuals, their feelings and family ties, and receive a different response from our patients in return.

These differences must have their origins in the main point of contact between doctor and patient, namely the consultation. They account for a growing conviction among some general practitioners that the technique of interviewing patients as taught to medical students and junior hospital doctors by consultants is inappropriate to the needs of general practice.

The general practitioner, however, cannot afford to forget nor ignore the more formal interview of his hospital peers. There are many occasions when he needs this method, but, most frequently, general practice lends itself to a less formal approach. Our observations are frequently gleaned through an oblique view of the patient rather than from direct questioning and a seemingly idle chat can often do more to establish a patient's confidence than the most sophisticated of medicines.

'The specialist has his function, but, to him, we are merely banal examples of what he knows all about. The healer I trust is someone I've gossiped and drunk with before I call him to touch me.'

W. H. Auden

And again, a patient describing Dr Pickles said:

... '[He] doesn't just come in and out saying, "We'll send a bottle of medicine along." He stops and chats and gives confidence. That's what a lot of these old people want. You'd be surprised how much medicine ends up down the sink.'

J. Pemberton—*Will Pickles of Wensleydale*

For many reasons, therefore, the relationship that the GP has with his patients will differ from that of the specialist. The GP will deal with all medical problems, and often non-medical ones as well, and not just those restricted to one specialty. In contrast the narrow focus of the specialist can leave the patient with feelings of exasperation, and even resentment, particularly when the patient is suffering from a terminal illness.

Usually a specialist consultation will have a very definite structure, beginning with the acquisition and assimilation of information, followed by appropriate examination, investigation, diagnosis and treatment or advice. For the GP, information is gathered from numerous short consultations over many years. The accumulation of this sifted material adds to or modifies the GP's current assessment of the patient's health and tolerance of illness. To a trainee observer each separate interview may seem to have very little meaning, perhaps no more than that, say, obtained from reading a randomly chosen paragraph from a novel. It is only in the context of seeing the patient in several interviews and with several different symptoms, that one can begin to understand the problems in any depth.

Knowledge and understanding of the patient grow from a knowledge of the family and the home. Home visits invariably provide insight into problems seldom revealed in the surgery. Knowledge of the patient's relatives and an awareness of their ill-health often provide clues for the doctor that direct questions in a formal interview would fail to reveal. Furthermore, in general practice it is not always immediately apparent whom the doctor should treat, the patient presenting with the symptoms, or perhaps the patient's relative causing the problem.

Problem identification rather than diagnosis is a not infrequent aim of general practice, but this should not be used as an excuse for clinical carelessness. A doctor should always strive for the most precise diagnosis possible. In general practice, however, there is often no formal or explicit diagnosis to be made.

These are some of the differences between the task of the GP and that of the specialist. The relationship is different, the aims are different and, therefore, the consultation should be different.

Change in Emphasis

The past 30 years have seen a considerable shift in emphasis in the style of consultation. In the 1950s, after the flood gates of medical demand had been opened with the birth of the National Health Service in 1948, doctors were encouraged to keep a tight rein on their patients. Direct question and answer was considered to be the ideal technique. Avoidance of all unnecessary talk was thought essential. Lord Taylor, when describing the art of good general practice in 1954, advised: 'The doctor with the heavy work-load will do well to avoid all unnecessary talk with his patients. It is a high clinical skill to make patients express themselves adequately in the shortest possible time.' He also stated that: 'The primary purpose of contact between patient and doctor, namely the making of the correct medical diagnosis and the application of the correct treatment, must never be allowed to get lost in a flood of verbosity on either side.'

There are, of course, many doctors who would still offer this advice as being a prudent safeguard, arguing as Lord Taylor did that 'Saying too much is more dangerous than saying too little, and the doctor's first duty is still *primum non nocere.*' It is undoubtedly true that careless statements to the patient can give rise to a lot of needless worry. Nevertheless, it is also true that too little information breeds a fear of the unknown, which may be so easily dispelled by a single explanation. In any event, the patient has a right to know what ails him, if he so wishes, even if this causes him anguish.

A closed style of consulting, however, does provide many advantages. Interviews are easier to time and appointment systems are more easily maintained. Doctors who restrict themselves to the formal confines of medical diagnosis find that the method helps them to eliminate problems that are 'strictly non-medical'. Such doctors suffer less exasperation as they need not tolerate what they consider to be irrelevant chatter.

However, there are serious disadvantages. The risk of distorting the patient's story is very real. The overbearing doctor can force acceptance of symptoms on the more suggestible patient, who, in his eagerness to oblige, is willing to change his story to suit what he imagines the doctor wants to hear. This subsequent distortion of the history may become permanent as the patient's perceptions of his illness change when confronted by the greater 'knowledge of the doctor'. The original anxieties and ideas about his illness or the fears that his symptoms raise within him may never be revealed, and so never relieved by informed reassurance. In fact the doctor's attempts at reassurance based upon his own false assumptions rather than the patient's worries, may raise anxieties about other possible illnesses never before considered by the patient. Such a directive technique is not the only method of history taking, however, and, in recent years, the pendulum of medical opinion has swung to a freer and more open approach—a patient-orientated approach. This method was shown by Byrne and Long to be used only very infrequently, although four years before, in 1972, Lord Rosenheim was strongly advocating that the patient should be encouraged to tell his own story in his own words. He talked of ... 'the great value of an understanding and open approach to the patient, and the need to interpret and meet his unexpressed, and often hidden plea for help'.

The advantages of an open approach are clear. It is more satisfying to the patient who prefers to have his flow of thought uninterrupted. It is also less intimidating and allows the patient to relax and, in feeling less restrained, avoid withholding information that he thinks the doctor might not want to hear. In stress-related disorders this can be very important and may provide insight about a problem that the doctor would otherwise miss. There is also less tendency for the patient's story to be distorted either by the doctor or the patient. Thus a more truthful picture emerges, and so fewer irrelevant investigations should be performed.

Although better communication occurs, the method is not without drawbacks. The timing of the interview is less predictable and can cause considerable annoyance to those practitioners who like to keep a fastidious eye on the clock. It is also subject to some abuse by the more egocentric patients who are prone to indulge themselves in ceaseless and often irrelevant waffle. Such patients are fortunately not very common and are easily identified. They can either be dealt with using a more restrictive technique or perhaps, more interestingly, by discovering the causes of their need for such self indulgence.

This open approach will not suit all doctors and for that reason it is facile to promote it as being the ideal method. As with any relationship between two people preference will depend upon the personalities of the individuals concerned. The doctor must be sensitive to this, both in himself and in the patient, and adapt his style accordingly. Flexibility is essential.

Partners in Care

Whenever a patient goes to the doctor he is invariably seeking reassurance, and this can only be given satisfactorily when the doctor clearly appreciates what it is that worries the patient. Patients are often ignorant of medical information and frequently make muddled sense of what they do know. It may be misleading for the doctor to assume from the presenting symptoms that the patient is thinking along the same lines as himself as this may be far from the truth. Such false assumptions by the doctor may result in misleading explanations which confuse the patient and add to his worries.

Tuckett has repeatedly emphasized the importance of being aware of the patient's own ideas and describes it as the 'patient's explanatory model', a term that may be criticized as jargon, yet is of great significance. Without understanding this, the doctor's attempts at reassurance will often be inappropriate.

After telling his story, the patient usually hopes that the doctor will provide some sort of explanation of the symptoms, and a diagnosis if this is possible. Rather surprisingly, however, this expectation is seldom adequately met. Indeed many practitioners in the past have deliberately avoided any sort of explanation. Dr John Pickles, father of Will Pickles of Wensleydale, felt no obligation whatever to provide an explanation to his patients. He would say, referring to the persistent type of patient, 'If they ask me what's wrong with them, I say to them, that's my business. Do as I tell you and take your medicine and you'll get better.'

Few patients today would willingly tolerate this sort of approach. They are much more knowledgeable about medicine and health, and with encouragement from the doctor are more prepared to be involved in decisions about their own care. They are more interested in knowing what is happening to them during an illness, a change which has become especially apparent in the context of terminal illness. It is one of the duties of the doctor to inform his patient and correct any misconceptions that there may be about the symptoms. It is only through knowledge that reassurance has any lasting value.

Involvement of the patient has much to commend it. The patient suffers none of the indignity that invariably results from being treated by a patronizing doctor keen on maintaining his distance. As soon as the patient becomes a partner in his own care he is immediately motivated to co-operate with the doctor in the treatment. Charles Medawar argues that an informed and questioning patient is a better patient, providing both stimulus and safeguard to the doctor, and helps the doctor to resist his urge to reach for the prescription pad. In the frequently occurring situations where the option to prescribe medication is open to debate, the informed patient will frequently choose not to have a prescription. He prefers to get by with as few medicines as possible. Only those with unrealistic expectations of modern drugs insist on a prescription.

A questioning patient is also a cautious one, and caution provides an important safeguard to the practice of medicine. He also keeps the doctor mentally alert, and prevents him from becoming a victim of tedious routine.

Paradoxically, time spent on informing patients will often save further time by reducing the frequency with which those dissatisfied ones return.

Common Faults

Probably more errors are made in the practice of medicine by failure to take good account of the patient's story than by any other single factor. Tiredness and an indifferent mood would be accepted by most doctors as a source of error but, commoner by far, is the failure to elicit a clear history from the patient. The balance between encouraging a patient to give a free and uninterrupted account of his story and extracting precise details of his symptoms is a fine one. It is inevitably true that the skill of the doctor is more important than the technique he adopts. An open style should never be a licence to be unsystematic. Clarification by the patient with an economy of interference by the doctor are the desirable aims.

Another common fault is that of premature diagnosis. A doctor should restrain his urge to make hasty conclusions until he has allowed the patient to make clear his problems. A restricted focus by the doctor makes the false assumption that the patient has only one problem. For general practice in particular this is often far from the truth.

Lack of interest, unresponsiveness and an indifferent attitude will all compound the doctor's tendency to error. Friendliness and genuine concern are, therefore, important qualities. They provide both a safeguard to good practice and a relaxed atmosphere for the patient.

Maguire and Rutter have discused these common faults in considerable detail, and indicate how medical students may improve their style of interviewing by close attention to the type of questions used.

Aims

It is likely that all doctors have received some sort of basic training in the art of history taking. Apart from brief intervals at medical school, our technique is rarely scrutinized. Even in final and postgraduate examinations our methods remain untested and unchallenged; only our findings and conclusions are put to the test. More emphasis is placed upon how we present case histories than the manner in which we elicited them. Could we as a profession be any more culpable than this? All doctors would agree that the consultation and, in particular, the history is the most important aspect of medical practice, and yet we assume that by the time a medical student reaches his final examination he has achieved an acceptable expertise in this area of his training. Byrne and Long's (1976) transcriptions of GP consultations suggest that this may have been a rash assumption.

In the first edition of this book, *Partners in Care* (1986), I suggested that the RCGP could provide a lead by incorporating some form of scrutiny of a candidate's ability to consult into its membership examination. This is now to be realized, not only within the MRCGP examination, but in the Summative Assessment of all GP Registrars. Clearly it has become widely accepted by teachers of general practice, that consultation skills and technique are valuable parameters by which we judge each other.

The aim of this book, therefore, is to encourage the doctor to reflect upon his own style of consultation. It is principally directed at GP Registrars who are still developing their technique, but I hope that it will be of some interest to established practitioners and make them question some of the things they do and have taken for granted. It will deal with the various parts of the consultation in the sequence in which they would logically be expected to occur. In reality, however, there are many problems in general practice which require more than one interview, and so the following sequence is frequently disrupted or altered:

1 The expectations that both doctor and patient have of each other, and the preparations they both make before the interview.
2 The welcome: during which the doctor establishes a relationship with a new patient, or renews it with a familiar one.
3 The patient's story: during which the doctor attempts to discover the reason for the patient's visit.
4 Partners in care: the doctor discovers the patient's own ideas and fears about his symptoms. The patient reveals the direction in which he wishes the doctor to focus his attention in the hope of being reassured. The patient also expresses his expectations of treatment.
5 Physical examination: the doctor pays close attention to both the physical signs he seeks to elicit and to the patient's thoughts about his examination.
6 Examination of the emotions: can listening cure? An account of the value, basis and technique of psychotherapy in general practice.
7 Personalities and problems: as an appendix to examining the patient's emotions, I have added this chapter which draws attention to difficulties that may arise because of personality problems of the patient.
8 Character unfolding: The doctor's personality. I have added this new chapter in the light of experience drawn from watching numerous video consultations. The last decade has provided much teaching material about the way doctors behave towards patients. Much of this is a reflection of the doctor's personality. This chapter

deals with how his own personality affects the relationship between himself and the patient, the understanding they have of each other, and the subsequent outcome of the consultation.

9   The illusion of objectivity: the doctor–patient relationship. The only way we can understand each other is through our own personality. The lens through which we view others is peculiar to 'us'. The assessment of personality is always subjective and depends upon the relationship between observer and observed. This is just as true for the doctor–patient relationship as for any other.

10 Simple explanations: the doctor declares his own opinion, and provides the patient with a simple explanation. He may use simple metaphors to explain difficult medical concepts. Finally, the doctor offers the patient a choice of options of management.

11 The farewell: termination of the interview and a possible invitation for a further consultation.

12 Video assessment.

13 Conclusions.

The past decade has witnessed a considerable improvement in the teaching of consultation techniques. The widespread use of video recording has facilitated this development and provided some of the best ever teaching material available for trainers in general practice. So convinced of this benefit are those responsible for the training and assessment of the new generation of young doctors that they have decided to include obligatory video assessment in their final Summative Assessment. This is to be a nationally standardized level of competence, and so far as is possible, it will be objective. GP Registrars will have to satisfy the assessors of their ability to consult before they can become principals.

Summative Assessment will be based upon four parameters:

a   MCQ to test knowledge and problem solving.

b   An audit which will be an original piece of work designed and carried out by the GP Registrar.

c   The video assessment.

d   GP Trainer's Report. This is a list of skills and attitudes, each with a declared minimum standard asking the trainer to state the basis on which he judged the GP Registrar to be of a satisfactory standard or otherwise.

The Video Assessment

The GP Registrar will be required to submit for assessment a two-hour long tape of consecutive consultations on standard VHS format with an incorporated timer device, or alternatively a clock, visible in the background. This is to try and ensure that the consultations so taped are consecutive and not edited. Patients who refuse consent to be video recorded must be accounted for in the accompanying log book. The tape should contain about twelve of the registrar's own consultations together with the written log of each, in which the candidate describes how easy or difficult they were. He should offer some relevant background information about the patient, and he is also invited to give some idea of whether or not he considers the patient's needs were fulfilled.

Each tape will be marked independently by two assessors who will focus upon the basic outcome. The assessors will be looking primarily for evidence of minimal acceptable competence in order to pass the candidate as adequate. However, the following elements to the consultation will be marked on a scale of 1 to 6 (6 being excellent, 5 good, 4 competent, 3 bare pass, 2 possible refer, 1 refer for further assessment). These elements are:

1   Listening—How well does the doctor listen and identify the patient's problems, and realize the reasons for his attendance?

2   Action—Whether the doctor appropriately manages and/or investigates the problem, and seeks help when necessary by referral to a colleague or consultant.

3   Insight/understanding—Whether the doctor demonstrates in his log book that he understands the process and outcome of the consultation. He should explain his actions, and identify any shortcoming. Background information should also be included.

4   Error—The presence of a major error which could lead to harm, or a series of minor errors causing the patient's inconvenience will result in the candidate being referred for further review.

In the case of the candidate's performance being considered unsatisfactory by one or other of the assessors, the tape will pass through the following sequence of steps:

1   It will be discussed with the Trainer and VTS Course Organizer. If they are both satisfied with the candidate, the tape may be passed.

2   If considered still doubtful, the tape will then be seen by two more external assessors.

3   If the candidate is still considered to be doubtful, the tape is then seen by the Regional Adviser, who will review it together with the Trainer and possibly a nominee of the candidate (e.g. a colleague, or representative from the LMC etc.)

Making such a long video recording will inevitably arouse in most candidates considerable apprehension, but with a little forethought and preparation it may not be too daunting. In fact, the experience can be enjoyable and is certainly likely to be instructive.

Recording one's self provides one of the best opportunities for self-teaching, because the tapes can be viewed time and again. Incidents, which at the time were previously overlooked, can take on greater significance. Far from being trivial, there are occasional fleeting moments within a consultation that can be of immense focal importance and, if picked up at the time, offer both patient and doctor a whole new insight into the problem. If missed, the opportunity may be lost for good.

One of the main aims of this new addition, therefore, is to offer the GP Registrar some helpful advice about recording his surgery consultations on video tape. I hope that in achieving this, the common pitfalls of making such a recording will be avoided.

Taped interviews, audiovisual recordings and role play have all been introduced into medical training within the last decade. Most established doctors, however, will not have experienced these innovations and may be sceptical of their value. Nevertheless, we probably all have a curiosity about our colleagues and how they practise, but our only common source of feedback about them, at present, is from occasional, vociferous and dissatisfied patients who have either willingly left or been removed from the list of a doctor, about whom the patients are now critical. Not surprisingly this biased group is not treated with much credibility by the medical profession.

To be a 'fly on the wall' during a colleague's consultation, is, I suspect, a secret desire of us all, and perhaps we would have a great deal to learn from such a possibility. It is for this reason that Byrne and Long's transcriptions and more recently, Jonathan Gathorne-Hardy's study about *Doctors* (1984) hold so much fascination. We have all evolved our method of consulting by trial and error. It becomes fixed only when we are satisfied or cease to think about what we do. The purpose of this book will have been fulfilled if it stirs the pool of dissatisfaction and prompts the conjecture that things might be different.

Chapter 2

Great Expectations

Symptoms alone do not persuade the patient to go to the doctor, for as many patients with symptoms decide not to seek medical help as those who do (Tuckett, 1976). Nor is the decision to seek help an indication of the severity of the symptoms for, as all doctors know, many patients have trivial symptoms, and many people with symptoms of potentially serious disease ignore them.

A patient's decision to go to the doctor is not so simple as it might appear. It is complicated by many factors, including the patient's personality, the thoughts he has about his symptoms, and his tolerance of them. It is also dependent upon his experience of previous consultations, the relationship he has with his doctor, the approachability and attitudes of his doctor, the pressure placed upon him by friends and relations, his experience of illness in others, and the sense he makes of medical information.

Having made his decision, a patient will inevitably have certain expectations which he hopes will be satisfied by the consultation. It is almost as important for the doctor to be aware of these expectations as to be able to diagnose his patients' illnesses.

A patient may visit his GP for many reasons other than to have his symptoms diagnosed. He may want reassurance, or to discuss his personal problems, yet, at the same time, he may offer misleading symptoms; he may have been worried by someone; he may come to renew his prescription, or to discuss changing his medication; he may want time off from work, or to persuade the doctor to agree with some line of action that the patient has already taken.

Although one might expect a consultation between doctor and patient to have a common objective, namely, that of diagnosing and treating the patient's ailments, and thereby to demonstrate cooperation between two people, such cooperation is often lacking. In fact many consultations are hot beds of mutual misunderstanding, discord, manipulation and even conflict (Freidson, 1962; Bloom, 1963; Stimson and Webb, 1975). The reasons for this are numerous, but ultimately culminate in the widely differing expectations that both doctor and patient have of the consultation.

The extent to which both doctor and patient are satisfied with a consultation depends upon the degree to which their expectations of each other are met. What are these expectations and how may a doctor prepare himself for a more harmonious interview?

The Patient's Perceptions

Patients are invariably apprehensive about going to the doctor. This is not solely as a consequence of a fear of what unpleasant illnesses will be diagnosed, but also to a feeling of uncertainty about the appropriateness of their visit. People do not always know whether or not they are ill, or whether they are sufficiently unwell to trouble the doctor. For advice and support, they may seek the opinions of others, who often worsen their fears. This third party may be well intentioned and offer good advice, but relatives in particular may frequently feel the burden of concealed guilt, and to avoid any accusation of neglect will bully the patient into going to the doctor's surgery. Their guilt may be felt so acutely, as to cause them to demand an urgent home visit, often at a weekend, much to the embarrassment of the patient, and annoyance to the doctor.

Conversations with others may distort and exaggerate the history and result in the patient presenting to the doctor when he himself may otherwise have ignored his symptoms, at least until later. This exaggeration may result from anxiety generated by the opinions of friends or from a desire to justify his visit to the doctor. In general, the greater the patient's uncertainty, the greater will be the influence of others, and the more likely will be the distortion of the history.

A fear that symptoms may be considered as trivial by the doctor, and dismissed as a waste of time, is also very common. This is inevitably affected by the doctor's manner and will be exacerbated by unfriendliness and an unwelcoming attitude. Trying not to bother the doctor

... even the wearing of a white coat is an obvious barrier to communication.

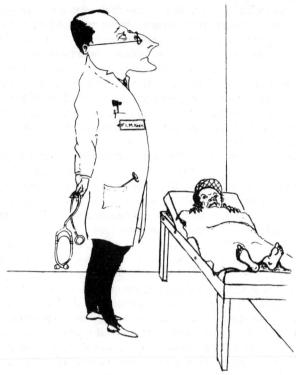

unnecessarily may not always be easy, for it is often not clear to the patient whether his problems warrant medical attention. Indeed, patients are frequently encouraged by the medical profession not to neglect early symptoms lest they be the herald of serious disease.

This underlying feeling of uncertainty and apprehension is compounded by fear of the diagnosis, of investigations, hospital referral, possible operations and worst of all of incurable disease. Moreover, all of these may be exaggerated by numerous other worries, many of which are within the realm of the doctor to dispel.

An unsympathetic attitude, an irritable mood, a clipped style of speech, an impatient manner, and even the wearing of a white coat are all obvious barriers to communication. Some doctors, who are guilty of this, may of course be unaware of their faults, but many feel that without these barriers they would lose the only restraints they have upon their patients. So, although the doctor is in a position to relieve his patient's fear, by his own defensive attitude and by his attempt to constrain the patient, he may in fact do the opposite.

Anxiety frequently causes the patient also to be defensive. He worries about being labelled as a time waster and deals with it by exaggerating his symptoms; he may even become belligerent and aggressive in order to justify his visit. Defences like this have provided many doctors with the idea that, if allowed, their patients would pour forth a torrent of relentless verbiage, but in reality this is far from the truth. Not all patients will respond to these barriers of restraint by becoming vociferous, and many will sit passively, quietly resentful of the doctor and exasperated by their own apparent submission. In such circumstances even though the consultation may proceed, any worthwhile communication ceases.

Much of this anxiety can be so easily relieved with a little consideration by the doctor, and yet the doctor's own apprehensions about the patient often result in failure. It is this mutual wariness and mistrust which lie behind the regrettable findings of Byrne and Long in 1976, namely, that the aim of most general practitioners is to usher the patient out of the surgery as quickly as possible.

Although the attitudes of doctors have the greatest effect on patients' anxieties, other factors should not be forgotten. Unaccommodating receptionists, rigid appointment systems, unwelcoming waiting rooms, and impersonal methods of calling patients into the consultation room all discourage, intimidate and lead to dissatisfaction, which rapidly spreads through the waiting room conversations of discontented patients.

Austere and clinical premises, sophisticated equipment, computers, video display units, buzzers, flashing lights, and plastic discs to indicate the sequence of patients, may reassure the doctor of his efficiency, yet frequently distance him from his patients. In medicine there is rarely any substitute for a sympathetic relationship between doctor and patient, and nothing should be allowed to hinder this.

The Doctor's Dilemma

Those doctors who have adopted an open style of interviewing know that the duration of their consultations is slightly less predictable and generally slightly longer, but they are also aware that having to tolerate a patient's self-indulgent chatter is a comparative rarity.

Most doctors aim to practise safe medicine and are genuinely concerned that a loss of restraining influences upon patients will confuse the history and subsequently impair safety. The doctors who advocate the removal of these restraints, however, maintain that the history will be less distorted and more truthful. Each doctor must resolve this dilemma for himself, for no single style will suit all doctors, nor all patients. The doctor should, however, be willing to try to improve whatever techniques he feels capable of using.

How else may the general practitioner prepare himself for the consultation? From his awareness of the source of patients' anxieties he can do a great deal to generate a feeling of welcome within the practice. It is his responsibility to see that the reception area runs smoothly. Care should be taken when interviewing future receptionists not only to be certain that they possess suitable qualities, but also to ensure that they are compatible with the other receptionists already employed. As a group they are not particularly well rewarded in financial terms and the doctor would do well to spend time in supporting them and listening to their grumbles. They should be included in practice meetings and encouraged to take an active role in practice organization. Contentment and a feeling of commitment do much to engender goodwill and cooperation, which will influence their management of the patients.

Receptionists have a difficult job and frequently suffer the abuse of irate patients. When things go wrong, it is the doctor's duty to know about it and to remedy the situation. Martin (1983) has written a guide to the selection and training of receptionists, and it is important for trainee GPs to have an early awareness of the difficulties that receptionists face.

Attention to the state of the practice premises and to the waiting room in particular are also important considerations. Patients will frequently spend more time in the waiting room than in the consulting room. It should, therefore, be a welcoming place conducive to relaxation. The decor should be restful and reflect a sensitivity to the feelings of the patients, many of whom will be ill, of course. Provision of toys and books for children will be appreciated by the harassed parent, as will suitable magazines for adults.

In many health centres and larger group practices, complicated systems exist to indicate to the patient his position on the doctor's surgery list. For example, on arrival at many such centres, patients report to the reception desk and are checked against the list of patients booked for the various doctors. They are given a plastic tab which is coloured to indicate the doctor with whom they are booked and who has a surgery door of the same colour. The tab is also numbered to indicate the sequence of patients. When the doctor wants the next patient to come in he pushes a button on his desk which is wired to a panel of coloured lights in the waiting room. The appropriate coloured bulb lights up, providing the stimulus for the next patient to proceed to the doctor after he has hung up his numbered tab on a matching coloured hook.

Such a remote control method of calling the patients into the surgery is probably unavoidable for most health centres because of their size and design and despite initial confusion, most patients rapidly adapt to it. It also provides the patient with the advantage of knowing how many patients are waiting to see the doctor ahead of him.

However, it is more satisfactory if the doctor comes out and calls the next patient by name. Complicated systems place a barrier between patient and doctor and serve to regiment and depersonalise the patient, which is surely opposed to the aim of general practice.

Just as important as the waiting room is the arrangement and decor of the consulting room. This should be to the mutual satisfaction of both doctor and patient. The arrangement of furniture and, in particular, the relative positions of doctor, patient and desk have a significant effect upon the emotional distances between doctor and patient (Ward and Stein, 1975; Short, 1980). Many doctors prefer to distance themselves from their patients by placing the desk as a barrier between them, which serves to reduce the emotional threat of contact. Those wishing to develop a more friendly relationship with their patients however, will place the desk to one side or even discard it altogether. Whatever arrangement is eventually chosen, it should feel natural and comfortable to both doctor and patient. This will of course depend upon the personality of the doctor who should be aware that an inappropriate arrangement will exaggerate the discomfort of the patient, and heighten the tensions between them.

How Many Patients and How Much Time?

The average number of patients on a general practitioner's list has been gradually falling since the beginning of the National Health Service in 1948. There is no accepted ideal list size and attempts to estimate it have been entirely frustrated (Butler, 1980). The reasons for this lie in the wide variety of practices, and the uniqueness of each doctor; comparability is almost impossible.

Nevertheless, there is fairly clear evidence that the more patients a doctor has on his list, the lower is his consultation rate per thousand patients, although the time he devotes to each consultation does not seem to be altered. Furthermore, doctors with larger lists express more frustration and dissatisfaction with the quality of their work than those with smaller lists.

Until there are clear national guidelines, each doctor will have to make his own decision about list size. This will, no doubt, be based upon financial considerations, but it should also involve the type of practice and his need for job satisfaction. The style of consultation and the relationship he wishes to develop with his patients will depend very much upon the time that he is prepared to spend with them. A schedule of appointments can only be satisfactorily resolved after careful attention to this problem (Howie, 1984).

From his own experience, which should be subject to frequent personal review, the doctor will know how many patients he can comfortably see in a surgery before becoming adversely affected by fatigue and irritability. Because he has an obligation to provide adequate time for each consultation and to provide sufficient appointments and surgeries to cope with the demand, he should be able to estimate the number of patients with whom he can reasonably cope. The only unknown factor in this calculation is the annual consultation rate per patient. Since this varies widely from practice to practice, the new GP will find the national average consultation rate of 3.7 a suitable guide with which to start.

For example:
   A GP with 2000 patients on his list and an average consultation rate of 3.7 per year will have 7400 consultations per year. Omitting Bank Holidays and assuming his partners or a locum see his patients when he is on vacation, this will average at 145 consultations per week
or
   An average of 7 surgeries of 21 patients per surgery.

Unless the other figures in the calculation are compromised, fewer surgeries per week must result in longer sessions. Attempts at squeezing more patients into existing fixed surgery times lead to inadequate numbers of appointments or inadequate consultation times.
   A doctor should provide adequate surgery time to fulfil his patients' needs and also to maintain or improve his own standards of service. He must also decide upon the duration of each appointment.
   It is illogical to assume that all patients require the same amount of time for each consultation. They express themselves with varying facility and present with a wide variety of problems. A fixed appointment system is inappropriate to the needs of general practice and only causes dissatisfaction in the patient and frustration for the doctor. It is also inevitable that, until the patient presents his problems to the doctor, the time needed for the consultation cannot be assessed. Some patients may be dealt with adequately in as little as 2–3 minutes, whereas many patients need 7–10 minutes and some much longer.
   Byrne and Long (1976) observed that most doctors had difficulty keeping to their appointment systems. Some were found to be consistently delayed in the earlier part of their surgeries and then managed to catch up by reducing the length of their later consultations. This attempt to speed up when behind schedule is probably widespread but is best avoided. Providing briefer consultations to patients who have waited longer to see the doctor is not only illogical but unfair and may lead to errors of management, as well as to resentment in the patient.

Appointment time		Patient and problem	Real consultation time (minutes)	Waiting time (minutes)
9.00 am	RS	Adult male, asthma	10	0
9.05	LB	Girl, hay fever and mild asthma	8	5
9.10	JS	Boy, eczema	10	8
9.15	NS	Girl, catarrhal otitis	10	13
9.20	VB	Girl, mild hayfever	5	18
9.25		GAP		
9.30		GAP		
9.35	WG	Woman, breast lump ?carcinoma. Referral	10	8
9.40	PM	Failed to attend		
9.45	MP	Man, diarrhoea and vomiting now ceased. Private certificate.	3	8
9.55		GAP		
10.00	VT	Woman, coil check one week after insertion	3	0
10.05	DA	Woman, depression— now fully recovered. Last of many visits	4	0
10.10	ER	Man, migraine	9	0
10.15	CS	Man, ear wash out	4	4
10.20	CA	Woman, mild hay fever. Seeing her again with child in afternoon	3	3
10.25		GAP		
10.30–11.00	NP	Woman, severe depression and phobias. Psychotherapy	45	0
11.05	AB	Woman, rheumatoid arthritis on penicillamine. Recurrent anaemia	25	15

Total length of surgery 2 hours 29 minutes

The longest wait was for patient VB — 18 minutes
5 of the 15 patients had no wait at all
The average consultation time was approximately — 10 minutes
The average waiting time was — 5.5 minutes

The usual duration of a GP consultation is about 6 minutes, but the range probably extends from 2 minutes to one hour. Clearly, very long appointments are best booked in advance and placed either at the end of a list, or at times other than ordinary surgeries. Hoping to provide an ideal and flexible system which prevents the patient from waiting is unrealistic, but this should not discourage the doctor from trying to organize a system which is fair to both the patient and himself. Many doctors book patients at intervals shorter than they can manage in the hope of not having to wait themselves, should they have some quick consultations during the earlier part of the surgery.

On the other hand, a growing number of GPs favour extending the average consultation time to 10 minutes but, in answer to this, there are many situations where the patient can be dealt with more than adequately in less time. A suitable compromise to this dilemma would be to book appointments at 5-minute intervals and to leave gaps of between 5–10 minutes every half an hour or as appropriate. These gaps can be lengthened or shortened, or inserted more or less frequently according to how well the doctor copes.

An example of a fairly typical surgery of mine in June 1984 is given on page 19.

Whatever choices are made within such a framework, the emphasis should be on flexibility. If, in practice, patients are found to be waiting unreasonably long periods of time, then more gaps should be allowed until this is remedied. The system allows for differences in patients' problems and variation in doctors' styles and must be constantly re-appraised.

It is also incumbent upon the doctor either to delay filling later appointments, or to have an open ended arrangement or some other alternative, to enable him to cater for emergencies. Frequent discussion with the receptionists will reveal any difficulties they may have in providing appointments, and constant vigilance for signs of patient dissatisfaction is a prudent safeguard. In any event, most patients are reasonable and are aware of the difficulties involved, as well as appreciative of any attempts to reduce their waiting time.

It is probably true to say that most people are resigned to wait provided they receive an adequate consultation time and satisfactory quality of care. They know that their doctor is busy and if he is not, they will probably be mistrustful of him.

In conclusion therefore, a doctor should pay careful heed to the needs of his patients before ever he sees them in the surgery. Patients are often well aware of the efforts made on their behalf to provide more comfortable surroundings, and better consultation times. An overall atmosphere of welcome and consideration is quickly acknowledged by the patients and invariably passed on to others in day-to-day conversation. Contented surgery staff usually convey their satisfaction to the patients and vice versa. However, the doctor should guard against complacency and keep a constant watch for signs of dissatisfaction among his patients.

Chapter 3

Welcome

... 'It is easy to acquire the bad habit of completing notes about the previous case at the crucial moment when the newcomer should be welcomed. The patient ... may be embarrassed by not knowing to whom he is speaking, and accordingly appropriate introductions should be made .... At the outset the doctor should do the talking while the patient adapts himself to the situation. Initial remarks should be about impersonal matters; a minute or so can be spent with profit in this way to help eliminate any preliminary diffidence. Any impression of hurry on the doctor's part must be avoided.'

J. G. Macleod—*Clinical Examination*

Regrettably the initial offer of welcome to the patient may be anything but welcoming, and indeed, on some occasions barely conceals the doctor's feelings of irritation and even hostility. Usually, however, it follows a set routine which varies little from patient to patient, and perhaps reflects the lack of importance placed upon this aspect of the consultation. Nevertheless, first impressions are usually long lasting and, with a little thought, the doctor can do much to foster good will and generate confidence.

We have already seen how the patient's first impressions of his visit to the doctor will be affected by the behaviour and attitude of the receptionists. We have also seen how these impressions will be modified during the time in the waiting room, through casual conversations with other patients and the attempts made by the staff to provide pleasant and comfortable surroundings.

The GP's first contact with the patient, therefore, should provide the opportunity to consolidate this already favourable impression. It will not be achieved, however, if the introduction is marred by misunderstanding, impatience and irritability.

To get off to a good start, it is important to be sure of the patient's name and to avoid any mistaken identity, especially when dealing with anyone having a common surname. If, when he wishes to see the next patient, the doctor goes to the waiting room and calls him by name, the chance of such confusion will be reduced. Buzzers and other remote-control systems do not have this advantage, so identity must be established when the patient confronts the doctor. In most instances the doctor will recognize the patient, but not infrequently may fail to recall the name and may have to ask. More unfortunate still is the situation where the doctor mistakenly thinks he recognizes the patient as someone familiar, and yet confuses him with another patient whose notes have been mistakenly provided by the receptionist. Such errors when discovered late in the interview may cause much consternation in the patient and embarrassment to the doctor.

How a doctor greets a patient is very much a part of his personality, but a simple acknowledgement of the patient's presence is the very least he should show. I recall a video recording of a real consultation during which the doctor scarcely raised his head from the desk or stopped writing. Even the handing of the prescription was performed in a dismissive manner with eyes averted from the patient. Clearly any useful human contact was lacking and the concept of 'doctor being the best cure' rendered totally meaningless.

Greeting the patient by name, rising from the chair when the patient enters, shaking his hand, indicating where he should sit, and even introducing himself to new patients, all convey a feeling of welcome and help to remove any constraints of anxiety from the patient. Whatever his manner of greeting, the doctor should try to be natural and friendly, and refrain from patronizing behaviour or obsequiousness. This offer of welcome should also be extended to relatives and friends accompanying the patient.

While acknowledging that the next patient has entered the consulting room, it is preferable for the doctor to have finished writing in the previous patient's notes, so that his full attention may be paid to the new arrival. This avoids instilling in the patient any sense of haste and allows the doctor the opportunity of considering any initial impressions that the patient's entrance might make. The time saved in making notes while the next patient is entering the consulting room is minimal, and hardly worth the disadvantages that result.

For those doctors who use computerized records, it is even more important to have finished typing in the previous patient's notes, and to have erased them from the screen before the next patient enters. Failure to do so may cause embarrassment and is certainly a breach of confidence.

Because the VDU screen is usually visible to the patient, it is even more important from the outset to establish the patient's identity correctly. To omit doing this can lead, not only to a breach of confidence and the doctor's entry being recorded in the wrong notes, but to the prescription being typed and handed to the patient with the wrong name and address. If this is subsequently discovered by the patient, it may cause considerable consternation and may even result in an official complaint.

It is vitally important, therefore, with every consultation not to get off to a bad start. The offer of welcome and firm establishment of the patient's correct identity can be done with emphasis, care and good humour without seeming over pedantic. The patient will at least appreciate the doctor's carefulness, and any resulting disquiet will have been avoided.

With new patients it is better to avoid launching into immediate statements about rules and regulations, which only case alienation. It is much more profitable to take the opportunity of making a few friendly enquiries about his past health, his family, his occupation, his previous address and the reasons for his recent move.

The manner of greeting a patient, therefore, can be greatly improved with a few simple considerations. Furthermore, by introducing a little variety the doctor may help to prevent an atmosphere of routine and convey a more personal emphasis to each interview. For the doctor a consultation will be one of many, but for the patient it is a more singular event. Evidence suggests, however, that we are influenced more by our own feelings than by those of the patient, and in consequence our manner of greeting follows an almost rigid pattern. This routine may stifle any intended warmth in the welcome, and the doctor should try to avoid it.

When a patient is late for an appointment, most doctors would expect an apology or an explanation. It is merely good manners for the doctor to do likewise, especially if the patient has been kept waiting for a long time. The usual reason for a delay to patients is a consequence of earlier appointments running unpredictably overtime. Though the doctor cannot altogether be blamed for this, he should at least offer an explanation, of course avoiding any breach of confidence. After all, the doctor's intention is mainly to demonstrate his awareness that the patient's time is also valuable, and to diffuse any feelings of exasperation in the patient before the interview begins.

Chapter 4

Listening with Sympathy

'In any consultation there are normally two parties—the doctor and the patient. The doctor has special skills and experience which may well be the key component of that consultation. It is wise to remember that the patient too has a unique pattern of knowledge and experience and that any consultation is made up of a mixture of the patient and the doctor.'

P. S. Byrne and B. E. L. Long—*Doctors Talking to Patients*

The Patient's History

Doubtless every doctor has memories of having made some astute diagnoses and is encouraged by these. Such feelings of satisfaction, however, are rarely shared by the patients, who have to bear the anxiety of such 'splendid' discoveries. In contrast, the gratitude that doctors do receive from patients frequently seems to be out of proportion to the benefits that they have obtained, a fact that is illustrated by the surprising number of 'thank you' letters from patients for whom little seems to have been achieved. The reason for this disparity rests on the different views that the doctor and patient have of their association. A patient's satisfaction will depend upon the fulfilment of his own expectations rather than those of the doctor.

As medical students, we were possibly all upset by our first encounter with illness. This was often exacerbated by the contrastingly detached way in which many of our teachers discussed their interesting cases. For them, clinical findings and laboratory data seemed to offer greater fascination than those considerations, which for the patients, were more important. Prolonged attention to medical details had restricted our instructors' focus and drawn their attention away from the patients' real problems. As medical students meeting patients for the first time, we were free from such distractions and more able to sympathize with their predicaments, a finding to which Knox *et al.* (1979) and Cole (1982) made reference when comparing histories taken by medical students with those by qualified doctors.

Of course it would be silly to suggest that attention to medical detail is a mere distraction and unimportant, but to ignore those aspects of the illness that the patient considers most relevant is a serious omission. A certain degree of emotional detachment is, if not essential, certainly useful. Having to listen frequently to patients' complaints can reduce a doctor's sensitivity and tolerance, and over-involvement may cause him considerable distress. For junior hospital doctors fear of such emotional commitment is rarely the reason for their frequently observed detachment. Rather, it is a lack of understanding due, most probably, to their immaturity and a preference for dealing with the more tangible and, for them, more interesting aspects of clinical medicine and laboratory data. This excuse can hardly be used by the family practitioner who ought to have both a greater experience of life and a closer human relationship with his patients. Nevertheless, there are still many general practitioners, who, through temperament and a reluctance to become emotionally involved, prefer to maintain their distance.

This, then, provides the basis for the variety of interview techniques that have been observed. All doctors begin learning their style of history-taking as medical students, and during their training adhere to well-documented guidelines. Later, through trial and error this style evolves into an almost automatic habit which bears only slight resemblance to the practice originally learned. Its evolution relies just as much, and possibly more, upon the doctor's needs as upon those of his patients.

Styles of Consultation

In 1976 Byrne and Long divided the spectrum of styles of consultation into four basic groups. These were not considered to be watertight compartments and, in reality, most doctors' styles range between the various boundaries. Though doctors usually prefer to operate within two such favoured groups, the particular style of a doctor refers to the overall pattern of his consultations, even though he will probably include a few questions which, on their own, would be classed as belonging to another group.

Figure 4.1 shows a model which demonstrates how these four basic styles differ from one another and how they relate to the doctor's willingness or reluctance to allow his patients to speak freely. Those doctors who wish to keep a tight rein on their patients, use direct closed questions which invite a similarly precise answer. They try to dominate the consultation and confine the patient's attention to those aspects which they consider relevant. Of this group Michael Balint said: 'The doctor who asks questions will get answers but little else.' His observation was aimed at criticizing those doctors who fail to listen to what their patients are really trying to say; thinking, instead, that they know better.

At the other end of the spectrum is the open style of consultation. This is a style ascribed to those who encourage patients to present their own history. It requires the doctor to listen and reflect upon what is said and to interrupt only to clarify a few relevant details. It encourages the

Fig. 4.1

Patient-centred
open-style →
→ Doctor-centred
closed-style

Use of Patient's Knowledge and Skill			Use of Doctor's Knowledge and Skill
Silence reflective listening	*Clarifying and interpreting*	*Analysing and probing*	*Gathering information*
Offering observation	Broad question	Direct question	Direct question
Encouraging	Clarifying	Correlational question	Closed question
Clarifying	Challenging	Placing events	Correlational question
Reflecting	Repeating for affirmation	Repeating for affirmation	Placing events
Using patient's ideas	Seeking patient's ideas	Suggesting	Summarising to close off
Seeking patient's ideas	Offering observation	Offering feeling	Suggesting self-answering questions
Indicating understanding	Concealed question placing events	Exploring	Reassuring
Using silence	Summarizing to open up	Broad question	Repeating for affirmation
			Justifying self-chastising

Reproduced by kind permission from *Doctors Talking to Patients* (1976) P. S. Byrne and B. E. L. Long, HMSO, London.

patient to take a much more active part in the consultation, and in this way the doctor hopes to gain greater cooperation.

Between these two limits of the spectrum lies a range of styles which is conveniently divided into two further groups, one involving analysis and probing, and the other of clarifying and interpreting. Byrne and Long observed that most doctors tend to interview using two styles adjacent within the spectrum. So, one who used a reflective style would also use clarification, and someone else, who preferred to gather information would also be likely to use the technique of analysing and probing. It would be unusual for a doctor who liked gathering facts also to use a reflective technique. Exceptions do exist, however, and most commonly occur with those who use a reflective style, the shift to information gathering being employed as a method of speeding up, or when faced with some difficulty in communication, such as a language problem, or with the deaf, or a person of limited intelligence.

Style is, of course, idiosyncratic, and to suggest that there is an ideal method to suit everyone would be false. Choice will depend upon the individual doctor and will be affected by the relationship he has with his patients. It seems likely that a doctor will use those techniques which he thinks suit him best, and any attempt to persuade him to change to another, which for him would be unsuitable, is likely to be unsuccessful.

Many established practitioners, however, seem to have developed their style by trial and error without much conscious thought, and have neither been aware of the effectiveness of their consultations, nor considered any alternative techniques. It was the aim of Byrne and Long to bring to doctors' attention the variety of styles available and to encourage us all to consider any possible improvements.

Flexibility of style provides several advantages because it allows doctors to modify their interviews to suit the needs and expectations of their patients and the particular illnesses with which they present. It also allows them to adjust the duration of their consultations when pressed for time.

A Closed Style—Directive and Doctor-centred

This style is closely related to the formal process of history-taking taught to medical students, and for this reason, not surprisingly, is still the most commonly used. It provides the safeguard that all doctors wish to retain, namely of ensuring that no serious organic problem should be overlooked. From this point of view it has much to commend it.

The doctor's aim is to confine the patient's attention to specific symptoms and their associations. For example, when a patient presents with pain, the doctor will consider it necessary to ask a series of questions to discover its site and distribution, its time of onset, its character, its

A Closed Style of Consultation: The doctor's aim is to confine his patient's attention to specific symptoms and their associations.

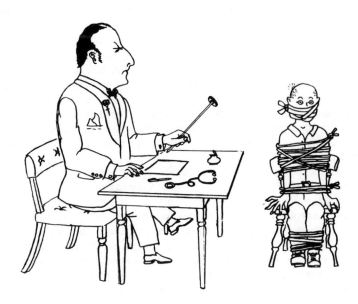

relationship with other symptoms, and so on. This is a technique which imposes a constraint upon the patient and involves a great deal of disciplined participation by the doctor. He talks frequently, asks direct and sometimes leading questions, interrupts the patient to establish points of detail and confines him to those matters which the doctor considers relevant.

It offers many attractions as well as the main one previously mentioned, namely of helping the doctor avoid errors of omission which might result in his failure to diagnose organic illness. It also allows him to cover a wide range of topics quickly and enables him to concentrate upon those he considers more important. Interviews are easier to time and appointment systems better regimented.

For specialists, whose patients have already been selected by general practitioners, it is arguably the preferred style of consultation, but for general practice it has many limitations. Patients frequently present with ill-defined symptoms, which may not represent organic illness, and are impossible to clarify, and more often than not relate to their feelings of unhappiness, resentment, and anxiety. The practitioner hoping to confine himself to dealing with organic problems will find these frequently recurring emotional problems tedious and time-wasting, and will be frustrated in his attempts to deal with them using this closed style. With this style, the doctor may learn much that is relevant to the diagnosis of a disease, but will appreciate little about the patient, his personality or his problems.

For the familiar situations in general practice a closed style involves the doctor in much effort for little return. In struggling to obtain a textbook history, he may miss valuable hints. Attempts by him to force clear, simple statements from reluctant patients probably exasperate both doctor and patient alike, and rarely present the doctor with a convincing diagnosis. Emotionally sensitive information, considered by patients to be of great importance, may be frequently ignored, causing much distress and resentment which will seriously erode any confidence the patient may have had in the doctor.

This not infrequent lack of perception and sensitivity was discussed by Fitton and Acheson in 1979, who recorded many transcripts of comments made by patients after their visits to the doctor. Feelings of frustration probably did cause the patients to exaggerate, but it was clear, from their point of view, that many consultations are a futile waste of time, a claim that is often echoed by doctors. In these instances the consultation must surely be at fault, and this may be because the style that was used was inappropriate.

A frequent complaint of doctors is that patients too often present with trivia. Trivial symptoms, however, may be the earliest sign of developing disease, and since the medical profession itself spends a great deal of time persuading the public not to delay seeking medical advice, it is hardly surprising that patients will often worry over simple problems (Hannay, 1979, 1980). Furthermore, trivial symptoms may also provide the excuse that patients who are emotionally upset need to seek help. A closed style of consultation does not provide the doctor with the easiest way of differentiating between symptoms which suggest early organic illness and those of an emotional origin. Only by allowing the patient to discuss his fears and the sense he makes of his symptoms on his own terms, will the doctor really understand the reasons for the patient's visit. Having a closed style for such situations causes both parties to be dissatisfied, often leading to dismissiveness by the doctor and bewilderment in the patient.

Open Style—Non-directive and Patient-centred

To the casual observer this style of consultation may seem unstructured and aimless because it relies upon the patient's initiative. The issues to be discussed are left open to the patient who is encouraged to talk freely and without much interruption. The clarity of the history will depend upon the patient, his intellect and medical knowledge, his perception and personality, and his mood. Of course the doctor must make allowances for any initial vagueness in the story, and later try to clear up any confusion about essential details.

On occasions patients ask questions of the doctor, and here it is sometimes more revealing to reflect the question back and ask the patient what he thinks. This is not an attempt to be evasive, but instead to reveal the patient's own thoughts and fears which may say much more about the reasons for his visit. However, the doctor does not sit passively while the patient makes all the effort, but rather he concentrates his attention upon listening and assimilating what the patient says.

The great attraction of this method arises from obtaining better co-operation with the patient, who is actively involved in sorting out his own problems. There is less emotional distance between doctor and patient and the patient feels none of the irritation which may occur when he is submitted to constant questioning which interrupts his train of thought. It is therefore invaluable in providing the doctor with information about his patient's thoughts and his response to problems. In fact it is the only satisfactory way of doing so, and as Macleod (1964) suggested, it is the style of choice when dealing with psychological problems. The frequency of such problems in general practice might suggest that this technique would be widespread but, paradoxically, Byrne and Long (1976) found it seldom used.

Giving the patient greater freedom of discussion avoids the distortion which may occur when the doctor is too rigid in his application of the closed style. Such over-enthusiastic constraint by the doctor may even cause the less resolute patient to admit to non-existent problems. An anxious patient under pressure from her doctor once remarked after the interview: 'When I got there and sat down, I didn't dare tell him ... in fact I told him a whole string of lies' (Stimson and Webb, 1975). In contrast, an open style encourages freer expression from the patient which releases him from the inhibitions caused by his anxiety. It allows him to digress and wander a little from the mainline of the story. This may seem wasteful of time but it is surprising how often flashes of insight about the patient's problems may occur to the doctor during such digressions. In any event, it invariably provides the basis for a closer human relationship between patient and doctor, for the simple reason that it appears to the patient more natural and less business-like than the constrained atmosphere of a closed style.

Though there are many doctors who would use a closed style when dealing with a depressed patient, mentally ticking off his various symptoms, as if to provide themselves with a diagnostic score, it is rarely a satisfactory way of talking about such problems in general practice. It only serves to alienate the patient who already feels isolated by his illness, and to categorize and dehumanize him when he most needs sympathy.

For the doctor who is unfamiliar with the open style of interview, its prospect may generate fears of congested surgeries and endless consultations. In practice this is far from the truth. Adoption of an open approach does not mean that the doctor abandons all control. Consultation times are more variable and those interviews with a psychological content generally take longer. Clearly it is impossible to hold a consultation using a reflective approach in 2 minutes flat, so allowances should be made in structuring appointments. Not all consultations, however, need be longer, and for many straightforward problems the allocation of time should be no different from that required for a directive approach.

Additional fears that the consultation will become haphazard and unsystematic are also groundless, for just as much sorting must be done in the doctor's mind. For the observer, of course, this is not obviously apparent. In avoiding the effort of constant questioning the doctor provides himself with time to consider what the patient is saying, to select more immediately relevant information, and store apparently less important points for retrieval later on. Such assimilation allows the doctor finally to select with economy a few pertinent questions and enables him to clarify some of the more relevant points. These questions will be aimed at resolving any ambiguities or idiosyncrasies of speech and obtaining precise dates or time intervals which might be important.

The Two-headed Model of Neighbour

As an aid to better understanding of the processes at work within the consultation, models are often used. Roger Neighbour, in his excellent book *The Inner Consultation* (1987), wrote a valuable précis of several such models, with particular reference to the consultation in General Practice. He likened their use to the role a transitional object has for a child.

A teddy bear or a favourite blanket often serves as a helpful link between the child's inner world and that outside. It enables the child to delineate itself from others. Whilst the comforting object comes from the outside world, it has so many of the child's own projections placed upon it, that it takes on a transitional role helping the child bridge the divide between itself and its outer environment.

Models provide a similar role, and according to Roger Neighbour are a useful way of introducing the student to consultation dynamics, which might otherwise be more difficult to understand. Furthermore, he introduces his own particular model of the Inner Consultation, which highlights the contribution of the right hemisphere of our brains to perceptual and abstract learning. The left hemisphere in most people is used for logical, systematic organization, the right for intuitive, spontaneous responses. Both heads, the 'Organizer' and the 'Responder', are equally important. Neighbour maintains that too many past models of the consultation have focused upon the functions of our left hemisphere at the expense of invaluable contributions from the right.

His model of two heads seeks to redress this imbalance. He provides a five-fingered list of checkpoints which he calls:

1 Connecting
2 Summarizing
3 Handing over
4 Safety netting
5 Housekeeping

1 *Connecting:* This involves not merely taking a history from the patient, but embraces the wider concept of establishing rapport, focusing upon intuitive hunches, and building up impressions from what is said and the gestures used by the patient to express it.

2 *Summarizing:* When the doctor feels he has obtained sufficient information, he offers the patient a summary or recapitulation of what has been presented. The patient may then ratify or modify whatever he feels is necessary to correct the doctor's impression.

3 *Handing over:* Before there can be any common ground between patient and doctor for the handing over of mutually shared ideas, the doctor must have a clear appreciation of, what Neighbour calls, the patient's framework. This includes the patient's knowledge, beliefs, attitudes, habits and opinions among other things. Only with this awareness will the doctor be able successfully to offer a management plan, to which the patient will adhere. Handing over, therefore, involves negotiating with and influencing the patient, before presenting advice that will be acceptable.

For example a mother may believe that all steroid sprays for asthmatic children are harmful. Before ever the GP can treat her asthmatic child, he should be aware of her opinion and deal with it. If he is ignorant of it and his intended treatment involves the use of inhaled steroids, the mother is unlikely to abide by the doctor's instructions.

4 *Safety netting:* When the doctor assesses the patient's problem, he should be also aware of any future possible developments. It would be better for the doctor to mention these at the time, especially if they are likely to affect the patient's confidence in him. For example, a GP treating a teenager with tonsillitis is well advised to caution him early on about the possibility of its being due to glandular fever. Simply to treat

the patient with penicillin, without doing so, runs the risk of the doctor losing credibility, when the penicillin fails to work.

5 *House keeping:* This refers to those aspects of the doctor's own well-being, which need constant attention, to enable him to work safely. All doctors have needs, which for one reason or another may be frustrated and cause stress. The doctor may be tired and need sleep, or feel inadequately trained in a particular aspect of his work about which the patient is now presenting. He may need to feel respected by his patients or just accepted as a caring physician, when in contrast, what he suspects they feel towards him is anything but respect. If he fails to be aware of these needs and to cater for them, his performance and subsequent safety may suffer.

Roger Neighbour details ways in which all these problems can be addressed, and refers frequently to the model he offers. Just as with the transitional object, so too with the model, once it has served its useful function it will be discarded but its influence remains.

Choice of Consulting Styles

As every consultation is a unique event no single style can be considered ideal, nevertheless, a great many consultations in general practice have a psychological bias and the use of an open style ought to be more common than it is. A doctor's ability to adapt his style to suit the situation will provide him with a certain advantage. An open approach is certainly the more satisfactory way of consulting patients who are emotionally upset, whereas when dealing with organic illness and when under pressure of time a more directive style allows the doctor to speed up, and yet still remain safe. This habit of speeding up is very common and is due, of course, to a desire to finish on time. Although understandable from the doctor's point of view, this habit is hardly satisfactory for the patient. To overcome this problem, especially if it occurs frequently, the doctor should reconsider his allocation of appointment times and be more adaptable with his style of consultation, using a restrictive approach at the appropriate opportunities. Conversely, on the occasions when he finds himself ahead of schedule, he might take the opportunity of adopting a more open approach and learn more about his patients.

Individual Personality

The competence of a doctor and the success of his relationship with his patients will depend upon his knowledge and skill, and his attitudes to his patients and the consultation. In general practice, more than any other branch of medicine, his success will also be dependent upon his natural

human qualities, his sensitivity and perception, his patience and understanding, his sympathy and his ability to listen. The extent to which
these qualities affect the interview was called by Balint, 'the doctor's
apostolic function'.

The degree of the doctor's sensitivity and perception will determine
the ease with which he is aware of the patient's unspoken feelings. The
familiar concept among GPs of a 'sixth sense' was described by Browne
and Freeling (1967) as an unexpressed feeling conveyed from patient to
doctor which provides him with some insight about the patient. Anger,
indignation, resentment, depression and anxiety are all readily transferred and are often feelings which the patient may avoid mentioning or
even simply deny. Emotions are often aroused in patients who are
worried during consultations. If the doctor is either unaware of such
feelings or tries to ignore those that are aroused within himself, he is
likely to miss valuable information. When the doctor senses these feelings, he should inquire about them, because they may lead him to the
main reason for the patient's visit. Patients have their own views about
where doctors' interests lie and often present with organic symptoms,
irrespective of whether these are significant to the problem. A patient
who is suffering from anxiety may have a tight sensation of discomfort
in the chest, and rather than go to the doctor complaining of anxiety,
often presents the symptom of discomfort which he considers more
acceptable to the doctor.

A doctor who is patient and understanding will encourage a different
response from his patients compared to a colleague who is not. This will
affect the content of his consultations and the willingness of his patients
to discuss more intimate problems. Patients often want to unburden
themselves of their more distressing problems, yet feel reluctant and
vulnerable about doing so to a doctor who is impatient and discouraging.
The doctor should be aware of these barriers in communication and try
to adjust his manner accordingly.

Sympathy

Sympathy is a blend of understanding, consideration and compassion. It
is a shared feeling which has been associated with the art of healing for
centuries, and for the general practitioner forms a vital part of his
practice. Despite the enormous improvements in medical care which
have rather distracted the public's attention in recent years, sympathy is
still one of the best ways in which a doctor can express his desire to help
the patient.

It is not just a passive feeling that arises from hearing of someone's
misfortune but plays an important instrumental role throughout the
consultation, encouraging the patient to be less reticent, and enabling

him to speak more easily about his distress. It may also provide considerable therapeutic rewards often exceeding those obtained from treatment with sophisticated medicines, yet its use is not without hazard.

Like any other instrument, the benefits of sympathy depend upon the skill with which it is employed and unfortunately, it is often misused. A common example of this is where there is a tacit agreement between a manipulative patient, who tries to evoke sympathy to gain an ally, and a doctor, who is reluctant to reveal his true opinions. Such collusion does provide mutual gain yet inevitably stagnates the relationship. There are many examples of this sort of behaviour.

Marital disharmony is a frequent problem among patients who present to the general practitioner. It is not uncommon for one of a married couple to try to gain the doctor's sympathy by giving a biased account, thereby hoping to obtain his collusion against the 'guilty' spouse. Should the doctor prefer to avoid confronting the patient with real insight about his behaviour, he effectively dodges his responsibilities by resorting to meaningless sympathy. The doctor gains from the superficial gratitude of the patient and by the abrupt termination of the consultation; the patient gains by having his opinions reaffirmed; yet no progress has been made and the opportunity for resolving the problems has been wasted.

Another less frequent example which occurs in general practice is that presented by the hypochondriacal patient who, for a variety of reasons, wishes to persuade the doctor to accept his symptoms as genuine. Such a patient may go to extraordinary lengths, inventing bizarre and occasionally progressive symptoms and often exchanging doctors in a relentless pursuit for acceptance and sympathy. Confronted with such patients as these, doctors often choose the line of least resistance and accept their demands, if only to rid themselves of the problem and avoid wasting more time. The problem rarely disappears, however, and the patient returns time and time gain for his regular 'dose of collusion'.

Sympathy can also be misplaced by being expressed prematurely, and this can have unfortunate repercussions on the doctor's relationship with his patient. Consider the example of a patient bereft of a relative, against whom he has deep yet concealed feelings of bitterness. The relative's death will invariably arouse a mixture of emotions: regret, guilt, frustrated resentment and perhaps even relief. If the doctor, in ignorance of his patient's feelings, assumes wrongly that their relationship had been a loving one, he may offer his condolences too profoundly and too soon, denying the patient the opportunity of expressing his real feelings. This may increase the patient's guilt and even cause him to redirect his resentment towards the doctor.

Friendliness

Another personal attribute which contributes to a better relationship with the patient is friendliness, which usually finds expression in casual conversation. One should not forget that patients are often genuinely interested in knowing a little about their doctor's personal life, his family and his interests. This should not be considered an intrusion into his privacy, but rather a desire for assurance that he is human, perhaps with problems similar to the patient's own. A casual chat often does more to generate confidence than a formal consultation. The general practitioner should be prepared for inquiries like this, and respond in a suitably friendly manner. If he wishes to avoid such intrusions, he should use tact and good humour to do so, to prevent tensions building up between himself and the patient.

Listening and Silence

Patience and the ability to listen constructively are fundamental to the art of history taking. So often do doctors miss important clues by jumping in too soon with their next question. Questions provide information but rarely insight, and yet the latter is often more revealing than information.

Listening requires a great deal of effort and concentration to sort out the relevance of various points and to consider their possible relationships. Silence can be used to positive effect by encouraging the more diffident patient to express himself in his own words, or to heighten the tension between doctor and patient where this may be useful. It provides the time in which to consider the problems and their implications and to reflect upon the various options open for management. A doctor who questions frequently spends much of his time thinking about his next question and less upon the answers he is given. Sympathy and listening when used with care and discretion form an important combination for any doctor, but particularly for a general practitioner.

Chapter 5

Partners in Care: A Shared Understanding

'If the doctor regards reducing patients' concern and giving care and reassurance to his patients as important, then he must make this appropriate by first establishing what his patients' concerns really are.'
David Pendleton *et al.*—*The Consultation: An Approach to Learning and Teaching*

Results from a survey by Ann Cartwright in 1967, indicated that over one-half of all general practitioners regard at least one-quarter of their consultations as trivial. A further review in 1981 showed that little had changed. Why is this and should anything be done about it?

The fact that doctors frequently consider that patients bother them with trivialities must reflect the differences in interpreting what is trivial; what is unimportant to the doctor may be extremely worrying to the patient. Interestingly, according to the same surveys, both doctors and patients seem to be aware of the existence of each other's points of view and yet little is done by either to try to bridge the gap between them. Very often patients who anticipate that the doctor will consider their symptoms to be of little importance, will still want to see him to obtain his reassurance. They will frequently begin by saying: 'I'm sorry to waste your time, but ....'. From such remarks it is plain to see that patients are willing to face the embarrassment of being considered time-wasters in the hope of settling their worries, which is surely an indication of how disturbing these anxieties are to the patient. It also shows how inappropriate it is for the doctor to complain that so many of his patients waste his time with trivia.

Unless doctors try to understand their patients' views and accept the reasons for their concern they will be unable to rid themselves of the feeling that patients often do waste their time, an idea which causes doctors so much unnecessary exasperation. However, this is not the only reason for encouraging patients to reveal their own ideas about their symptoms. Only by knowing what worries the patient, can the doctor begin to treat his problems properly. Unless he has a clear idea of how the patient views his symptoms, he will be unable to offer suitable reassurance and correct the misunderstandings the patient may have about medical information.

Reassurance

All too often reassurance lacks a firm footing. Unsupported, its efficacy may rest solely upon the doctor's authority and the patient's gullibility. Its duration is seldom more than ephemeral. Successful reassurance needs to be based upon mutual respect, common understanding and factual information. It is born from the consultation, but is conceived beforehand in the attitude and regard that the doctor and patient hold for each other. Respect is a hard earned commodity, yet one which is fragile and easily tarnished, so it is incumbent upon a doctor to try always to do his best, and to be seen to do so.

Concern for patients is manifest in so many different ways, not just from the doctor's own behaviour, but also, as we have seen, in those more distant aspects of the consultation, such as the manner of the receptionists, the atmosphere of the waiting room, and the time allocated for consultations. All provide the setting for good consultation. All these factors are essential for effective practice.

Thereafter it is the doctor's approachability and his willingness to explore those avenues of concern which the patient considers important, that prepare the way towards worthwhile reassurance. Educating the patient, correcting his misunderstandings, and providing him with a satisfactory explanation for his symptoms are the only sure means of fulfilling his need for peace of mind.

Ideas and Idiosyncrasies

Until recently, almost no attempt was made to encourage medical students to enquire about their patients' ideas and the sense they make of their symptoms. This probably accounts for the lack of emphasis and interest that today's established general practitioners place upon this aspect of the consultation. For hospital specialists, whose patients have already seen a doctor, it is perhaps understandable that they should ignore this, but for the general practitioner there is no such excuse. It is in fact a very important part of the patient's history as it reveals those particular worries that are special to him (Tuckett, 1976, 1982).

Not surprisingly the ideas that patients have about their symptoms are often quite different from those of the doctor. There are many reasons for this. Doctors base their hypotheses upon formal medical practice, but even so they also are influenced by other factors, some of which are not medical. The doctor's mood and temperament, the sort of relationship he has with the patient, and his previous experience with similar problems are some of the factors which influence his conclusions. Despite years of training such vagaries do still affect him, so it is scarcely surprising that patients display similar idiosyncrasies.

... the ideas that patients have about their symptoms are often quite different from those of the doctor.

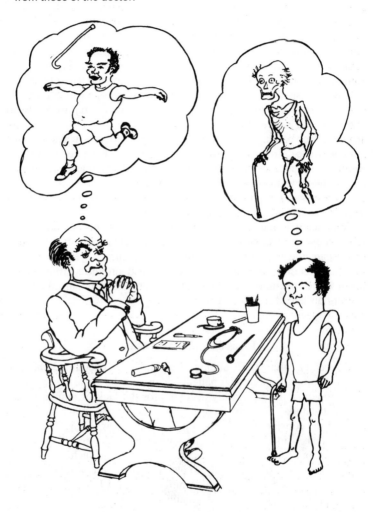

Patients do not have the benefit of sophisticated medical knowledge, yet they do try to make their own sense of available information. Sometimes this is muddled, but often it is surprisingly accurate. Like doctors, patients, too, are influenced by past experiences, either their own or that of friends and relatives, and their fears are certainly affected by their prevailing mood and their personality.

consultation, and have subsequently developed a profound respect for the huge variety which is the richness of general practice.

In another context, I should like to acknowledge my debt for the experience I gained in working alongside Alan Ruben, Regional Adviser for SE Thames and his Associate Advisers, Ben Perkins, Roger May, Ken Evans and Zoe Kenyon. Especially among this team I wish to thank David Armstrong, Reader in Medical Sociology at Guy's Hospital for his influence and academic stimulus, and for introducing me to videos which fuelled my growing interest in the way personality affects communication. It ultimately resulted in the chapter 'Character Unfolding: The Doctor's Personality'.

My thanks are also due to the following for permission to reproduce extracts from copyright material:

Regents of the University of California: *Empathy Revisited: The Process of Understanding People* (1959), by Fred Massarik and Irving R. Wechsler.

John Woodall: *Self Awareness* (1966) (personal communication).

Oxford Medical Publications: *The Consultation: An Approach to Learning and Teaching* (1984), by D. Pendelton *et al.*

Victor Gollancz Ltd, London: *Doctor! Doctor! An Insider's Guide to the Games Doctors Play* (1986) by Michael O'Donnell.

Barely a week before my publisher's deadline, I had the good fortune to bump into John Woodall, a retired GP and past Associate Adviser for SE Thames. He had been working on a short dissertation about self awareness, and he generously gave me a copy. Within an instant I recognized that it was what I had long been searching for. Our chance meeting resulted in the brief but important chapter The Illusion of Objectivity, and for that I would like to offer him my heartfelt thanks.

Whilst acknowledging the help of all concerned, I accept full responsibility for all the opinions expressed and for any misinterpretations I may have made from others work.

Finally, I should like to thank Sue Cover, the Librarian at the Kent and Canterbury Postgraduate Medical Centre and Natalia Watson and Norma Watson for typing additions to this second edition with speed and efficiency, and with remarkably good grace, given the time constraints placed upon them.

Acknowledgements
for the Second Edition

No doubt one of the greatest debts a teacher owes is to his pupils and their enthusiasm to learn. Education, particularly in a one-to-one relationship is reciprocal. For this reason I have much to thank my own GP Registrars, who all deserve mentioning by name: Vanessa Potter, Julie Fegent, Mike Goold, Gill Collier, Roz Waller, Zsuzsanna Russ, Jane Drouot, Hélène Armstrong, May Shiu Chan, Elaine Wylie, Helga Paul and Simon Wilson.

Without their influence and contribution to my own education, many of the ideas, particularly related to the way personality affects the consultation, would probably never have been realized.

Within the Canterbury and Thanet Vocational Training Schemes I have met some splendid young doctors, with whom it has been a real privilege to be associated. I owe them much gratitude and I shall watch their progress with keen interest. I regret that there are too many to mention by name here.

I should especially like to thank my Co-Course Organizer, John Semple, who has helped me in so many ways. Being such a naturally gifted organizer he has shouldered much of the burden that would otherwise have been mine, so allowing me to focus more of my attention on my main interest, namely teaching. Furthermore, through numerous conversations with John, I have gained a much greater insight about general practice, and have thoroughly enjoyed his company.

In this respect I should also like to express my thanks to Murray McGregor and Graham Field, Course Organizers from Thanet with whom John and I have shared many VTS workshops.

I should also like to take this opportunity to thank Tony Membrey, who succeeded me as Associate Regional Adviser and made cooperating with him a source of stimulation, interest and encouragement.

The Canterbury Trainer Workshop has also been a source of continuing support to me, as has the Kent Postgraduate Centre, and the Kent Institute of Medicine and Health Sciences at the University of Kent at Canterbury.

Within my own practice, my partners Henry Byrom, Madeleine Richardson, Bill Lloyd Hughes and Julie Fegent have and continue to have a profound influence on my professional life. I thank them for that and would like to acknowledge their support and tolerance of me. I have been very privileged to work with colleagues with such varying styles of

Earlier drafts were overburdened with too many references, which made it cumbersome, added little, and were counter to my intention. I have, therefore, deliberately excluded many of them, and have, thereby, risked being accused of presenting evidence which may seem anecdotal. I would like to assure the reader that this is not the case. As the book was written for GP Registrars rather than researchers in general practice, I hope this decision will not cause undue irritation and inconvenience. In an attempt to counterbalance this omission, and also to encourage further reading, I have added a few appropriate commentaries in the bibliography.

Summative Assessment is aimed at setting a basic level of competence in order to separate those doctors who would be safe general practitioners, from those who would not. My intention, however, is to provide candidates with the help required to attain the highest level of achievement in either Summative Assessment or the MRCGP Examination. This book, therefore, is designed to help all candidates with their video assessment, up to and including the level of Distinction at the MRCGP. Furthermore, by introducing many standard references and encouraging further reading about the consultation in general practice, I hope it will prove useful in other parts of the examinations.

Throughout the book I have kept to the male pronoun 'he'. This is for convenience and in almost all instances it could be substituted with 'she'. I trust my decision will cause no offence.

Finally, I should like to wish all those about to embark upon videorecording the same enjoyment and reward that I have gained in this exercise.

process. The left hemisphere, the Organizer, analyses thought in a linear rational manner using words and concepts, whilst the right, the Responder, reacts intuitively and perceptively with images, sensations and associations.

We are all different and it is pointless to try and impose a cloned ideal when the participants in the exercise are so very different. The disciplined aspects of our thought processes necessarily adopt the scientific code. This underpins our practice of medicine making it safe, but the responses of our right hemisphere are arguably equally important.

In the first edition, I wrote about the different aspects of patients' personalities and their influence upon clinical presentation. I have enlarged upon this in the second edition with further thoughts about doctors' personalities. With the advent of the video camera it has become possible to see exactly what happens between doctors and their patients during the consultation. Many of my earlier suspicions about the relationship between the doctor's character and the style of his consultation have been amply confirmed.

For this reason, in this new edition, I have added another chapter entitled, 'Character Unfolding: The Doctor's Personality'. I have written in greater detail about a few aspects of personality that affect the consultation, so that a young doctor on the threshold of his career might have an earlier insight about himself, and, through this awareness, be given an opportunity to modify the 'unfolding of his character'.

This is not intended to be a comprehensive description of all personality types but merely offers an introduction. Professional standards are important and should never be overlooked, but so, too, are the ways doctors listen and talk to their patients. After all, the relationship that a GP has with his patients, just as much as his professional skill, is the measure of his success.

Recently introduced regulations require all GP Registrars, who present themselves for Summative Assessment or the MRCGP Examination, to produce two hours of videorecording of their own consultations. This will inevitably cause much anxiety, and one of the main aims of this second edition is to help them with this task. Rather than being onerous, it can be enjoyable and is certainly instructive. Videorecording is probably one of the best ways in which a doctor may learn from himself. It has provided us with one of the most successful teaching aids this century.

In keeping with the simple themes of this book, I have tried to write in a way which, I hope, is easy and enjoyable to read. I have, therefore, avoided jargon, which is tiresome and unnecessary. Despite the comparative brevity of this book, it has been extensively researched, took over three years to complete and is based upon a wide source of medical and sociological literature.

Preface

In the first edition of my book, then entitled *Partners in Care*, I posed the question, 'What makes a good doctor?' As even the best of us is capable of indifferent practice at one time or other, I considered it more appropriate to ask, 'What makes a good consultation?'

The purpose of this book is to provoke young doctors into thinking about the various aspects of the consultation in the hope that they may reflect upon their own practice, and ultimately discover what for them is successful and what is not.

It would be reasonable to hope that with time, effort and application, improvement would draw us all nearer to our full potential, but in reality over the years many things get in the way. Tiredness, disinterest, dissatisfaction, overwork, irritability, anxiety and forgetfulness are just a few of the obstacles we GPs face in our working lives.

George Eliot in Middlemarch described this uncertainty through the development of one of her main characters, Dr Lydgate. He was one of the first surgeon-apothecaries of the early nineteenth century and the prototype of today's general practitioner. She wrote of Lydgate on the threshold of his career:

'He was certainly a happy fellow at this time: to be seven-and-twenty, without any fixed vices, with a generous resolution that his action should be beneficent, and with ideas in his brain that made life interesting …. He was at a starting point which makes many a man's career a fine subject for bettering … with all the possible thwartings and furtherings of circumstance, all the niceties of inward balance, by which a man swims and makes his point or else is carried headlong. The risk would remain, even with close knowledge of Lydgate's character; for character too is an unfolding. The man was still in the making, as much as the Middlemarch doctor and immortal discoverer, and there were both virtues and faults capable of shrinking or expanding.'

One of the fascinations of general practice is its variety: the variety of the patients, their illnesses and their presentations, and the doctors who treat them. Though the practice of medicine conforms to a standardized science, the art, the means by which we reach our diagnoses is anything but standardized.

Roger Neighbour in 1986 wrote in detail about the way our two cerebral hemispheres, right and left, fulfil two separate roles in this

Contents

Butterworth-Heinemann
Linacre House, Jordan Hill, Oxford OX2 8DP
A division of Reed Educational and Professional Publishing Ltd

℞ A member of the Reed Elsevier plc group

OXFORD   BOSTON   JOHANNESBURG
MELBOURNE   NEW DELHI   SINGAPORE

First published by William Heinemann as *Partners in Care* 1986
This edition published 1996

First edition © Peter Livesey 1986
Second edition © Reed Educational and Professional Publishing Ltd 1996

British Library Cataloguing in Publication Data
A catalogue record for this book is available from the British Library.

Library of Congress Cataloguing in Publication Data
A catalogue record for this book is available from the Library of Congress.

ISBN 0 7506 3130 9
(First edition ISBN 0 433 19600 9)

Typesetting by David Gregson Associates, Beccles, Suffolk
Printed and bound in Great Britain by Biddles Ltd, Guildford and King's Lynn

The GP Consultation
A Registrar's Guide

Peter G. Livesey

MD MBChB DObstRCOG

General Practitioner, Canterbury

Trainer and Course Organizer
Canterbury Vocational Training Scheme

Past Associate Regional Adviser in
General Practice for SE Thames
Member of the Executive Committee of the
Kent Institute of Medicine and Health Sciences (KIMHS)
at the University of Kent at Canterbury

Illustrations by the author

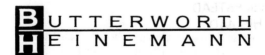

BUTTERWORTH
HEINEMANN

Attitudes

Many doctors still feel that it is their duty to obtain a clear and concise history, and would perhaps be concerned about spoiling their technique by being distracted by the patient's muddled ideas. Others no doubt hold fairly entrenched views about their role as diagnosticians and feel that patients should accept what they tell them. It is also likely that many patients accept this attitude from their doctors.

However, on the television, radio and in the newspapers, there is so much medical information now available that the idea of entrusting oneself completely to the hands of the medical profession is becoming anachronistic. Whether they want to or not, patients do know a good deal more about their bodies than they used to, and also are more aware of the shortcomings of doctors. Patients, who once would have been content to let the doctor get on with the job, are now less so, and there is a new generation who not only wish to express their own views but also wish to be involved with decisions about their treatment.

Though much health education is presented in the media, the only reliable source of personal contact for most people will be their general practitioners. It is part of his role to provide patients with the information that they require and to correct any mistaken ideas that they may have. The GP will not be able to do this satisfactorily unless he has the appropriate attitude and is willing to make himself approachable. He must first learn to encourage his patients to disclose their thoughts about their symptoms and to talk about their conclusions.

Initially, most patients will be diffident about revealing their ideas to their doctor, because of his superior knowledge. They will not wish to feel foolish by displaying their ignorance or by demonstrating their confused ideas. It is, therefore, most important that the doctor should put them at their ease and avoid any temptation to belittle them. When first making such enquiries, it will perhaps surprise many doctors to discover how much their patients know, and yet how often even seemingly knowledgeable patients become muddled. Medical terminology is a minefield even for medical students, so it is perhaps not surprising that patients frequently confuse terms. I have known people mix up names such as haemophilia with haemangioma, phlebitis with flea bites, erysipelas with syphilis, and cervical spondylosis with ankylosing spondylitis.

Such misunderstandings may be very amusing, but they also indicate the considerable anguish and unnecessary worry that some patients suffer. The patient who was told she had cervical spondylosis and thought she had ankylosing spondylitis had read a great number of disturbing facts about her disease and had spent several years worrying about her possible future life in a wheelchair. Similarly the mother of a child with a venous haemangioma had worried for over 10 years about the future crippling consequences of haemophilia, and was perplexed and upset that her child was not being regularly reviewed in a haemophiliac centre. Sadly, it is not rare to find that simple misunderstandings like these have caused patients years of anxiety.

Yet despite all this encouragement to involve patients in discussing their problems and making decisions about their management, there will always be some who reject this approach, and wish to remain in ignorance. Doctors should be aware of this also, and avoid being too enthusiastic in attempting to gain the patient's cooperation.

What We Need to Know About Patients' Ideas

Having established that patients do have thoughts about their symptoms, and that there is some value in discovering what these are, it is worth considering how best to use them. Pendleton *et al.* (1984) described in some detail how the GP may do this.

First, it is important to identify and outline the patient's ideas, and then to encourage him to enlarge upon them. There may have been many occasions in the past when the patient has suffered similar symptoms and yet not consulted his doctor, so it may be worth asking why he has decided to come on this particular occasion. It is also informative to inquire about his understanding of the problem. If, for example, a patient with chest pain thinks he may have angina, it is important to know what the patient understands by this condition, and especially how he thinks having such a condition could affect his general health.

People are concerned when they experience unpleasant symptoms and the anxiety caused by these will vary from person to person. It is important for a doctor to know a patient's particular worries and how he thinks his symptoms will affect his future way of life, for example his job prospects, whether he will still be allowed to drive, or whether the risks involved would prevent him from continuing his normal level of physical activity. Only by establishing the patient's concern can the doctor begin to reassure him. Without such information their discussions will often lead to misunderstandings.

In an earlier chapter we have seen how patients have certain expectations of the consultation. Some of these will relate specifically to the presenting problem. Without knowing what the patient expects of him, the doctor may unwittingly offer inappropriate help and advice. Much of his effort may be wasted because it is not recognized by the patient and, although the doctor may feel he is doing a good job, this will not be appreciated by the patient.

Lastly, it is important for the doctor to realize that symptoms do often have effects which, to the patient, may be more disruptive than the illness which caused them. Deterioration of physical faculties may often bring about a change in social circumstances and this may be the reason for the patient or his relatives to visit the doctor. In such instances it may be more suitable and more practical to try to improve the patient's social circumstances than to alleviate his symptoms.

Whatever the problem, the doctor can cope with it more effectively if he has a clear idea how his patient thinks about it and what his expectations are. Complicated investigations, medicines, advice and reassurance may all be misdirected and ultimately wasteful of resources. It is a disquieting thought that the vast amount of money wasted on medicines which are never taken may be mainly due to a failure of communication between doctor and patient.

Chapter 6

Say What You do: The Physical Examination

'[Many patients] appeared to set almost as much store on being examined as they did on being given a prescription.'
F. Fitton and H. W. K. Acheson—*The Doctor/Patient Relationship*

It is traditionally considered by the medical profession that an adequate history provides the diagnosis whereas physical examination merely confirms it. However, patients are usually unaware of this rule and often place greater importance upon being examined, even perhaps as much as upon being given a prescription (Fitton and Acheson, 1979). Certainly any advice, treatment or reassurance will have greater influence with the patient, when a thorough physical examination has been performed.

Yet, in general practice, there are many occasions when examination is unnecessary. There are also situations where examination is not performed either because the doctor is in a hurry, or because he feels that it would probably reveal very little useful information. In making this decision, however, he may fail to take account of the patient's expectations, and his omission may cast doubt in the patient's mind, leaving him with the worrying thought that his doctor did not do a thorough job.

The decision whether or not to examine is, of course, a professional one based upon the medical needs of the particular problem. Nevertheless, it is worthwhile considering the patient's own expectations as well as what is medically desirable. Doubt is hardly a sound basis for providing the patient with a credible explanation for his symptoms.

The methods of physical examination have been described in many textbooks, so I do not intend to repeat or elaborate upon them. Instead, I should like to consider the effects that the examination has upon the patient, for the doctor should not only possess the knowledge and skill to perform an examination properly, but also be aware of its effects which, from the patient's point of view, are probably just as important.

The Patient's Feelings

When a patient goes to the doctor he is often anxious. He may be afraid of what the doctor might discover or be worried about the significance of his symptoms and what changes in his life will result as a consequence of the diagnosis. He may also be concerned that his symptoms will be considered sufficiently serious to warrant a full medical examination and, therefore, being examined may confirm his fears. Conversely, he may be equally apprehensive that his doctor will not take him seriously enough to perform an examination. To be treated dismissively, if he feels he might have something serious, is upsetting and perplexing. The patient does not know whether to feel relieved that his doctor considers it trivial or annoyed that the GP does not seem to care enough.

Once the doctor has decided that an examination is warranted, the patient is both relieved and alarmed; relieved, that the doctor is taking the matter seriously enough to perform it, and yet alarmed, that his problem might not be simple and cannot be easily dismissed. Throughout the examination his worries will grow with the thought of what may be eventually revealed. To add further confusion to these mixed feelings, the patient may be baffled as parts of his body are examined that to him seem to have little or no relationship to his presenting complaint. He may be shocked or embarrassed by certain aspects of the examination or unable to stop himself from making frightening deductions by associating his symptoms with the various parts of himself being examined.

Some aspects of the examination may be particularly worrying. For example, symptoms of numbness or loss of power of a limb which result in the doctor paying close attention to the patient's eyes, head and muscular coordination may well convince him that his fears of a possible brain tumour are indeed justified. Alternatively, the patient may feel that those parts of his body that he associates with his symptoms are not receiving the attention they deserve, while the doctor seems far more interested, and perhaps even distracted, by other parts. This is common when the patient presents with a referred symptom. As a consequence he may even doubt the abilities of his doctor, which may cause alarm. Does the doctor really know what he is doing? Has he paid attention to what has been said?

Many such thoughts pass through the minds of patients. How, then, should doctors deal with the problem during the examination, and how may they best prevent the growth of unnecessary worry?

How to Earn the Patient's Trust

The best way to inspire confidence is to treat the patient's anxieties with the respect that the patient thinks they deserve. This means that, having previously asked the patient what thoughts he has about his own symptoms, the doctor must try to examine appropriately and keep the patient simply informed about what he is doing. So if, for example, the patient is worried about having a possible cancer, this must be explored, even though medically it might be an unlikely possibility. Perhaps in this respect general practice differs again from hospital medicine. Discussion about the patient's fears and about the links he makes between his symptoms and his conclusions are the first steps towards reassurance. Examination of the patient with consideration for his needs provides the means whereby reassurance will have some lasting value. Worrying conclusions must be openly discussed and shown to be incorrect before the patient can be adequately reassured. A dismissive attitude by the doctor is likely to make the patient feel foolish and resentful and will do nothing to alleviate his fears.

It is therefore important to involve the patient in his examination. By explaining briefly and simply what he is doing, the doctor will help to remove any bewilderment and inspire trust. In this way the patient will improve his awareness of what his doctor is trying to do and

If an examination is likely to be uncomfortable the doctor should be honest about it and warn the patient, but at the same time calm his anxiety by assuring him of the minimum of discomfort.

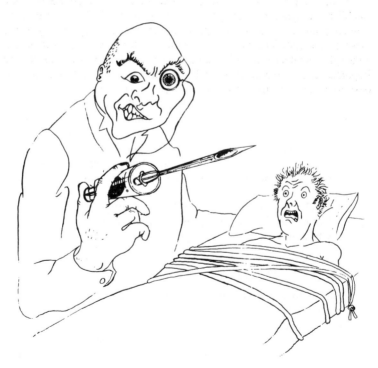

will also be better able to appreciate his thoroughness. No doubt he will still be worried about what may be discovered, but his doctor's concern and willingness to involve him will help dispel his apprehension and convince him of the reliability of any subsequent information and advice.

Taking the trouble to explain what he is doing is even more important during intrusive examinations, for although it may be routine for the doctor, to the patient it is not. Rectal and vaginal examinations, proctoscopy and venesection all require preliminary reassurance together with an explanation of what is involved and the reasons for performing it. If an examination is likely to be uncomfortable the doctor should be honest and warn the patient, but at the same time calm his anxiety by assuring him of the minimum of discomfort. If pain is caused the doctor should be aware of it and have the courtesy to offer a simple apology. By being conscious of the patient's predicament, the doctor generates confidence, reduces the patient's anxiety and, as a result, minimizes his discomfort. A caring attitude together with skill in performing examination procedures will be greatly appreciated by the patient and add to his feeling of trust.

Of course, the main purpose of the examination is to help the doctor establish a diagnosis. During the consultation he will have formulated some hypotheses. Examination provides him with the opportunity to put these to the test. The other considerations that have been discussed, although secondary to this, nevertheless have their own particular importance, and examination with regard to fulfilling all aims is both desirable and so easily achieved.

Chapter 7

The Story or the Analysis.
Can Listening Cure?

'The only death the spirit recognises is the denial of birth to that which strives to be born: those realities in ourselves that we have not allowed to live. The real ghost is a strange persistent beggar at a narrow door asking to be born; asking, again, again and again, for admission at the gateway of our lives.

Sir Laurens van der Post—*The Seed and the Sower*

'The hospital, where I went next morning, was a collection of bungalows, between the old and the new towns. It was kept by Franciscans. I made my way through a crowd of diseased Moors to the doctor's room. He was a layman, clean shaven, dressed in white, starched overalls. We spoke in French, and he told me Sebastian was in no danger, but quite unfit to travel. He had the grippe, with one lung slightly affected; he was very weak; he lacked resistance; what could one expect? He was an alcoholic. The doctor spoke dispassionately, almost brutally, with the relish men of science sometimes have for limiting themselves to inessentials, for pruning back their work to the point of sterility; but the bearded, barefooted brother in whose charge he put me, the man of no scientific pretensions who did the dirty jobs of the ward, had a different story.

' "He's so patient. Not like a young man at all. He lies there and never complains—and there is so much to complain of. We have no facilities. The government gives us what they can spare from the soldiers. And he is so kind. There is a poor German boy with a foot that will not heal and secondary syphilis, who comes here for treatment. Lord Flyte found him starving in Tangier and took him in and gave him a home. A real Samaritan." '

Evelyn Waugh—*Brideshead Revisited*

The judgement we make and our observations about people's behaviour depend upon a great many factors. Not least, our own experiences influence the sort of information we seek to obtain from patients and the impressions we form about them. Conclusions often reveal as much about the observer as the observed.

The formal discipline of history taking as learnt at medical school encourages the doctor to concentrate upon the details of individual symptoms rather than the overall story. For example with patients who are depressed, we are urged to inquire about interference with sleeping, early morning waking, loss of libido, loss of outside interest, loss of drive etc., and by assessing the severity of each symptom, make an assessment of their mental debility. Such regimented application might be useful within the confines of hospital psychiatry, but it is not the most appropriate method for general practice. The inexperienced doctor, preoccupied with making a diagnosis, and trying to fit patients into strict categories may easily be blinded by a list of symptoms and completely fail to understand what the patient is trying to say. All too often he may fix his attention upon his next question rather than listen to the patient's answer. In an attempt to reach a succinct conclusion we, too, may be 'guilty of pruning back to the point of sterility'. In general practice the 'different story' is often far more interesting, and revealing.

The obsession for slotting patients into neat diagnostic categories is, of course, understandable. A poorly understood problem is exasperating for both patient and doctor, whereas once the condition is diagnosed it is no longer idiosyncratic; it is a recognized manifestation of a common suffering for which there is usually a well tried form of treatment.

Misery, however, is not so easily categorized. Even though diagnostic groups such as acute anxiety stages and endogenous depression may be convenient terms of reference, they seldom help the doctor to understand his patient and almost invariably lead him to prescribe psychotropic drugs.

The tranquillizer boom started in the 1960s and met with the same meteoric rise in popularity as that experienced over a decade earlier with the advent of antibiotics. Why this took off so suddenly is probably more complicated than might at first appear. Tranquillizers were, of course, effective and worked quickly. People wanted them, just as groups of people, both past and present, have depended upon tobacco, alcohol, opium, and marijuana to induce relaxation. By contrast, tranquillizers seemed relatively safe, having been tested by the pharmaceutical industry and given official approval by the medical profession. They did not seem addictive in the way that narcotics and amphetamines were known to be, and they probably reflected a growing confidence in the benefits of the new therapeutic revolution.

Impatience among some doctors having to tolerate the complaints of neurotic patients, and exasperation in the face of an increasing problem, especially during the 1950s after the birth of the National Health Service, gave rise to the hope that such a panacea would work. In any case, a number of doctors may well have felt aggrieved that patients expected them to deal with their personal problems, problems which these doctors maintained were hardly medical and which most were ill-trained to handle. The optimism, therefore, that these psychotropic medicines generated, fired the enthusiasm of both doctor and patient alike. Yet regrettably this enthusiasm and a lack of caution led to eventual overprescription and abuse.

Not all the medical profession, however, were equally convinced by this trend and many notable exceptions, including G. M. Carstairs and Michael Balint were strongly advocating that general practitioners should listen to their patients rather than prescribe for them.

In 1963 Carstairs wrote:

> 'Perhaps nowhere in the contemporary society can be seen such clear evidence of the persistence of magical thinking as in the doctor's willingness to be persuaded (well, half persuaded) that the drug houses have the newly discovered elixir of life. In recent years extravagant hopes have been centred upon the psychotropic drugs, drugs which will relieve agitation and depression, and others which calm the turmoil of the acutely deranged. These drugs are often effective, if only for a time; but they have been used so intemperately that we still know remarkably little about their scope and limitations and their possible dangers; and yet they are being prescribed today in their millions. I do not wish to deny the help these drugs have brought to many seriously ill patients, but only to point out that when they are taken to relieve the emotional distress caused by problems of living they are merely anodyne, and offer no lasting solution.'

Twenty years later such advice has not gone unheeded and now, together with a growing public mistrust in the widespread use of psychotropic drugs, some doctors are setting aside their prescription pads, preferring, instead, to listen.

The Value of Listening

The last half century has witnessed a relentless growth in technology which, for all its undoubted advantages, has had a simultaneously dehumanizing effect on people's lives. Although modern medicine has certainly benefited from such advances, this has not been without cost. We have deceived ourselves with the illusion that for every problem there must a solution. In the context of human suffering this is far from the truth.

For the many who suffer and for whom no realistic solution can be provided, care, acceptance and understanding are often the only source of comfort. Our preoccupation with searching for a solution often distracts our attention from the one factor that is likely to be of benefit, a sympathetic ear.

Although patients who are incapacitated by their emotions may feel great relief when first treated with psychotropic drugs, they often have contrasting feelings of guilt and self reproach for not being able to cope without them, and sometimes also of resentment towards their doctor for dealing with their problems in such a superficial way. Since emotional problems are invariably seen by the person who suffers from them as being special and uniquely personal, it would seem more desirable to deal with them on a suitably personal basis. Whatever the final method of treatment, there is scarcely any excuse for not doing so during the interview. A psychiatric history which concentrates upon gathering information and listing symptoms is a poor substitute for listening to the whole story, which the patient will only tell when he is given time and encouragement.

An obvious further advantage of such an approach is the great sense of relief that is often felt by the patient after he has told his story. If, however, he is not allowed to express this adequately, he is more likely to suffer frustration, anger and even despair.

There is perhaps within us all a natural resistance to the idea that emotions can cause physical symptoms. Yet anyone who has suffered bereavement will have experienced a variety of real physical sensations which could not be dismissed as imaginary, and anyone who has felt anxiety about a forthcoming examination will, no doubt, have suffered from the real physical discomfort which usually accompanies it.

Few would deny the existence of such mechanisms, yet many patients, when ill and confronted with the possible explanation that their undiagnosed symptoms could have an emotional basis, initially reject the idea as unlikely. Perhaps it is part of repressing intolerable feelings that we also reject their link with physical symptoms. In some way our physical symptoms are preferable to the emotions we need to conceal, and may serve the purpose of enabling us to avoid facing our emotional conflict.

Of course, not all patients deny their feelings, and those who remain aware of them may wish to discuss them with their doctor. Regrettably, however, some doctors deal with such patients by attempting to confine the discussion to their physical symptoms. If the doctor will not accept their emotional symptoms, patients quickly learn to stop offering them, and instead concentrate upon their physical ailments, no matter how trivial these may be. It is, therefore, very important that if a patient chooses to discuss his emotional problem with a doctor, the doctor should respond appropriately, otherwise his consultations will degenerate to a discourse about mere trivialities.

Listening can provide consolation and comfort. This is the premise upon which all supportive psychotherapy and counselling are based. The doctor requires sensitivity and patience and, contrary to the meaning implicit in this recently popular term, 'counselling', should avoid giving advice. Listening may also cure. Psychoanalysis through emotional re-education seeks to do just this.

A general practitioner, of course, could not hope to practise extensive psychoanalysis because of the enormous commitment needed. Nevertheless, with a modest investment of time it is perhaps surprising how much may be achieved. Michael Balint maintained that the general practitioner was in an ideal situation to provide this service, and succeeded in persuading many doctors throughout the world that this was a worthwhile pursuit.

The doctor's aim is to have a greater understanding of his patient and to offer him some insight into his emotional turmoil, but to achieve this, he must have some understanding of the ways in which emotions may be aroused and the manner in which they can result in physical symptoms.

The Basis of Emotions and Emotional Symptoms

There are many theories about emotional behaviour and it is worthwhile for a general practitioner to become familiar with at least some of those that are generally accepted. The object of this section is not to discuss in detail all the various ideas but rather to present a view about the fundamental forces which lie behind our emotions and reactions, and to encourage those who are interested to delve deeper.

Compared with many living forms on earth *Homo sapiens* is very much a newcomer. Although we are different from our mammalian ancestors in the degree of our intellectual ability and in our capacity to communicate with each other, we are all still subject to the more primitive drives of our forebears. This animal inheritance is deeply rooted within us and only thinly disguised by our intellectual advancement. Survival of the herd, self-preservation and perpetuation of the species are all inextricably linked and form the most basic and powerful driving force in the higher groups of animals. To these ends man has so far been supremely successful.

For the benefit of the herd each member must compete with his fellows to ensure both strong leadership and a successful new generation. This rivalry, however, causes a wariness of each other and a profound feeling of insecurity, which forms a basis for many of our emotions (Fig. 7.1).

The difference between man's behaviour and that of other mammals, however, lies in the way he expresses his instincts. Being intellectually advanced, our primitive impulses are 'sublimated' in more recently acceptable forms of social behaviour. We are no longer necessarily expected to fight each other in order to prove who is the stronger, but we

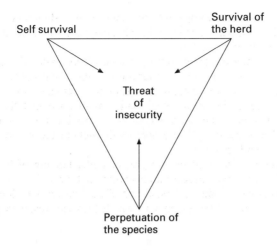

Fig. 7.1

have inherited these same determining biological impulses. We see our fellow as a competitor, fear him as a rival, and often try to conceal our insecurity from everyone, sometimes even from ourselves. Indeed almost to prove to ourselves that we do not feel insecure we often devise elaborate methods of self-deception.

Many of us endeavour to be successful at sport, or strive for academic distinction. Sometimes we try to acquire material wealth or perhaps seek fame and sometimes even notoriety. Some individuals wear uniforms or robes of office, others rely upon or hide behind the respect commanded by a chosen job or profession. Many take a pride in their appearance even though they may choose to give the impression of studied neglect. Others crave so much for superiority and the 'adulation of the crowd' that they abandon restraint, and become almost obsessed with their image, and in a sense become slaves to their own narcissism. Of course, we are concerned not merely with the visual appearance of our disguises but rather by the way we imagine others judge our character and our personality. No matter what image we create, we all conceal our real uncertainty beneath such disguises and the variety of the masks we contrive is enormous. But, although we may feel more secure through these disguises, we are also vulnerable because of them. Should we lack sufficient resilience, and our disguises be unadaptable, events may catch us out.

Without exception we are all born with this legacy of insecurity which not only make us wary of others, but also instills in us a desire to prove

No matter what image we create, we all conceal our real uncertainty beneath such disguises and the variety of the masks we contrive is enormous.

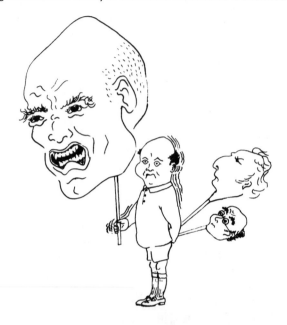

our worth. Although we wish to compete with each other and need to be self-assertive, we also recognize our dependence on and our obligation to the herd, which often takes precedence over our own individual needs. Self-interest and our responsibility to others are frequently incompatible, yet our fear of social rejection and the guilt and shame that invariably accompany it will often curb our selfish instincts. Such simultaneous and yet diametrically opposed driving forces suggest a possible basis for ambivalance, a term which describes the coexistence of conflicting emotions in one person.

The means we adopt to overcome our insecurity will depend upon our personalities, our natural qualities and the success or failure of our attempts to do so. Yet despite such wide variation, these primitive forces are the basic spur for all our actions and are probably expressed most transparently in the games we play.

Although it is possible to understand what lies behind our emotional feelings, our behaviour is far from predictable. Many of our emotions are unpleasant and painful, and so present a threat to our peace of mind. In order to maintain some stability, we devise ways of lessening their effect. What are these and how do we try to cope with unwanted feelings?

How Do We Cope with Disturbing Emotions?

An important factor in the development of emotional problems is our widespread reluctance to acknowledge them. Not only are we unwilling to talk about our feelings because of what may be revealed about our ability to cope, but we often deny their existence even to ourselves. For example, it is far more common for people to cling to their misunderstandings about each other than to say openly what they really feel. Why this is so, and why we should feel so embarrassed about being frank is often excused on the grounds of politeness, but there is another reason for our reserve and this is the fear of revealing our true selves, our faults and our weaknesses.

We try to cope with feelings that threaten to disturb our emotional stability in a variety of ways. We may attempt to deceive ourselves by rationalization, maintaining that what has caused our upset is after all unimportant and trivial. We may try to 'laugh things off', and indeed, humour is a common and remarkably successful way of diffusing tense situations. Voluntary suppression, distraction and subconscious repression all perform similar roles with variable but usually only temporary success. Sometimes we escape into fantasy to protect ourselves from the pain of the real world. At other times we produce neurotic behaviour and illnesses for, as we have already seen, it would appear that sometimes we find even illness more acceptable than admitting the existence of painful emotions. Perhaps the least successful of all our attempts to maintain emotional stability is the way we resort to dulling our senses with alcohol, tobacco and tranquillizers. Yet none of these methods is completely successful and our problems frequently re-emerge, often in other ways, and sometimes long after our original emotional distress has been forgotten.

Talking about one's problems and thereby achieving a greater self-awareness is one way of resolving our turmoil, but overcoming our apprehension and displaying our weaknesses is always an uncomfortable experience, and can occasionally precipitate a severe emotional crisis. The development of such a situation should be of great concern to anyone involved in psychotherapy, as the disturbance which may result can drive the patient towards suicide.

Psychotherapy is a method which provides no easy solutions and the therapist should avoid offering falsely optimistic claims of success. Yet it does give the patient often the only opportunity to discuss his real feelings. It also offers him a very close relationship with someone who is prepared to listen, to understand, and to accept his problems.

How Should We Listen?

At first this question may seem facile, perhaps even absurd, but to listen without unnecessary interruption or without asking leading questions is considerably more difficult than might be imagined. Just to listen requires considerable patience and attentiveness. So often are we inclined to interrupt, offer advice and explanations, or finish the patient's sentence when perhaps his flow of thought seems to have halted. We frequently prefer to reassure the patient about his worries rather than consider the implication of his search for reassurance. We always select the information given to us by the patient, often unfortunately, forgetting or ignoring what at the time seems irrelevant.

In an earlier chapter we discussed the pros and cons of the different styles of history taking, and saw how, when dealing with emotional problems, the urge to gather information is best restrained. Its use should be confined to obtaining such details as the patient's family history and the timing of events; beyond this an open style is desirable.

As well as style, the provision of appointments is also an important consideration. When talking about embarrassing problems, patients must not feel rushed. Clearly the duration of a consultation cannot be unlimited, yet a reasonable length of time needs to be provided. The amount, of course, will depend upon how much the doctor is able or prepared to spend, but it seems unlikely that really sensitive issues can be adequately discussed in much less than half an hour. A crowded waiting room will only make the patient feel uneasy, so ideally such appointments should be allocated either at the end of a surgery or perhaps better still at a completely separate time.

When providing supportive psychotherapy it is also important for the doctor to resist giving advice. Should he offer a plan of action which later results in failure, he will have to face the embarrassment of being blamed and his suggestions, if followed, may even cause the patient lasting misery. Balint described the potential risks involved if a doctor tries to offer what he considers to be sound 'common sense'. When dealing with problems about human relationships there are seldom any easy solutions.

Psychotherapy in general practice aims to be mainly supportive and the frequency and number of consultations that could be considered adequate will depend very much upon the degree and duration of the patient's distress. Supportive therapy offers the patient a sympathetic hearing in the hope of relieving his emotional tensions. It does not attempt to change him, or to re-educate him emotionally as does analytical therapy.

To some extent all consultations are supportive even if they focus exclusively upon organic diagnoses. For many problems needing supportive care, a single interview will often be enough, whereas with insoluble problems, consultations may continue for a lifetime. All general practitioners have some such seemingly dependent patients, and from time to time we must all wonder what we achieve for them, and why they return with such monotonous regularity. In general, they seem to prefer a neurotic way of life and have no apparent inclination to change it. For them, despite obvious disadvantages, neurotic symptoms are preferable to the repressed emotions which cause them. Such patients have an almost insatiable appetite for talking about their problems, no matter how inattentively the doctor may listen. To them even sympathy can sometimes seem unnecessary, and insight certainly unwanted.

When considering the advisability of using an analytical approach such patients are best excluded. In supportive therapy, on the other hand, selection is invariably done by the patient. It is he who chooses the doctor to pour out his troubles to and it is the doctor's duty to accept this role no matter how ill-suited he may feel. It usually takes the patient considerable courage to come and speak about his anxieties and the least the doctor can do is to conceal his own embarrassment and feelings of inadequacy. He should avoid getting flustered and try instead to consider the patient's predicament rather than his own. To let the patient down by immediately deciding that he is unqualified and incompetent to deal with such matters is upsetting and dispiriting to the patient.

Everyone can provide supportive therapy. It needs no special medical knowledge, but simply requires patience, and the willingness to listen and respond with kindness. The act of listening provides the patient with immense relief and gives the doctor a great advantage in the process of healing.

Analytical Psychotherapy

The general practitioner comes to know his patients and their families over several years and sometimes through many unhappy and stressful events. He is able, at first hand, to observe the relationships between the various members of a family, and to watch them grow and develop. In this respect he is in a unique professional position. Furthermore, by being aware of his own reactions to the patient's relatives, he may discover clues about his patients' reactions to them. His position, therefore, gives him a great advantage. Yet paradoxically, this relationship with his patients may also be a barrier to communicating with them. For example, there will be occasions when the doctor has made such close friendships with his patients that inquiry about sensitive issues might cause them considerable embarrassment. For each situation the GP must be aware of his own relationship with his patients and try to be

58 · The GP Consultation: A Registrar's Guide

sensitive to their feelings. After all, psychotherapy when handled tactlessly may be nothing more than a gross intrusion of the patient's privacy.

Because of his workload and because he is not a specialist, the GP is not in a position to offer complete formal psychoanalysis. Nevertheless, the insight he can provide may be rewarding to both doctor and patient alike. Yet this service is time-consuming and does require the doctor to be selective, towards both his patients and their problems. In this respect as we have seen, it is different from supportive therapy, where the patient is the one who exercises choice.

In selecting patients for analytical therapy, the doctor should observe a few simple rules. The problem should not seem so intractable as to offer no reasonable hope of improvement. The patient should be reasonably perceptive and intelligent, willing to participate, and have demonstrated his past ability to adapt to some of the stressful situations that he has already experienced during his life. The relationship between patient and doctor should be free from antagonism and mistrust, and neither should feel overawed by the other. Both should feel able to discuss any problem that may arise and both should trust in the honesty of each other.

As an additional role, it is advisable to have some simple and realistic aim which should be clearly discussed with the patient in the early stages of therapy. Otherwise consultations may drift aimlessly, and ultimately achieve very little. The purpose of therapy may be simply to introduce the patient to some of the emotions that in the past he has repressed or denied, and so provide him with a better understanding about himself. It may be to convince the patient about the psychological basis of his symptoms and so avoid referring him for yet another specialist's opinion, which, in such situations, is often arranged in the faint hope of convincing the patient that nothing organic has been overlooked. It may be to offer him an explanation for some of the bewildering feelings or neurotic symptoms that he is experiencing; or, together with supportive therapy, it may be used to stop the patient relying on tranquillizers. Whatever the aim, the doctor should bear in mind that by offering the patient a simple and realistic horizon, his expectations are not falsely raised. Furthermore, by offering a plan, he will be able to contain the total duration of therapy to a reasonable length. It is also advisable from time to time during the course of consultations to assess with the patient the current state of progress and the nearness he has come to achieving his aims.

In this way, the concern and reluctance that some patients feel towards the termination of their therapy is reduced and the state of dependency upon the doctor minimized.

It is impossible in a short space to describe in any satisfactory detail the various techniques of analytical psychotherapy. In any event, the subject has been exhaustively described in many specialist textbooks. However, for those unfamiliar with the method, it is hoped the following few paragraphs will provide a simple introduction and some understanding of the principles involved.

We have already seen how conflicting instincts often cause us to experience simultaneous and yet widely differing emotions, and this forms the basis of ambivalent feelings. In many instances we are aware of this ambivalence, and accept it with resignation, but occasionally events arise which are so disturbing that some of the feelings provoked are intolerable. These are repressed, leaving us aware of only those we find acceptable. However, repression is not achieved without cost, and this is generally believed to be the beginning of a neurosis.

To reveal the painful emotion which led to such repression, the doctor needs to direct his patient's attention to the events in his life just before the start of his neurosis. A history of the patient's behaviour and of his family relationships much before this event is certainly useful in providing information about his reactions in other situations, but it will not explain the source of the neurosis. So, while it is important for the doctor to listen to all that the patient says, he should pay particular attention to those feelings closely associated with events which led to his problem.

The doctor should also encourage his patient to consider any other feelings that he might have experienced had he not repressed them and which because of his repression he still finds difficult to acknowledge. Such suggestions may seem to the patient initially absurd, irritating, and perhaps even upsetting, and make him react accordingly. Because these reactions may represent stifled feelings from the patient's past, the doctor must keep a watchful eye for any signs of such reactions. The more disconcerting the suggestion, the greater will be the patient's emotional response. For a variety of reasons, however, the patient may be reluctant to admit to such reactions, so it is up to the doctor to bring them into the open and encourage his patients not only to acknowledge their presence, but also to talk about them honestly. On noticing the patient's response, the doctor might say: 'What we have been talking about seems to have upset you. Would you like to tell me about it?' Often, in this way, the patient's long forgotten feelings are reawakened in the form of a transferred reaction directed against the doctor. This is called 'transference' and is generally accepted as being one of the most important aspects of psychoanalysis. If the feelings so evoked pass unnoticed by the doctor, they may have only fleeting expression before they are once again repressed. The patient will have no clear idea what caused him to react the way he did, and the opportunity for exposing them will have been lost.

The purpose of analytical therapy, therefore, is not only to provide the patient with insight about the presence of his repressed emotions and the source of his neurosis, but also to help him experience those emotions which he previously refused to acknowledge, and thereby help him to come to terms with them.

A Note of Caution

A patient's reactions in the surgery do not necessarily relate to the event that the doctor is exploring, and it is important that the doctor should be aware of this and not jump to erroneous conclusions. Only by careful and sensitive questioning will such mistakes be avoided.

As with any consultation the doctor should beware of prematurely focusing his attention upon hasty speculations. It is better simply to listen and offer no conclusions than to rush at false and inappropriate ones. Theories about the basis of emotional behaviour provide the doctor with a framework to help him understand his patients' reactions, but they should not be used as a model for providing an easy and oversimplified analysis of the problem.

It is also advisable to avoid shortcuts either by trying to hurry the patient or by appearing to be a step ahead of him, offering him conclusions that he is not yet ready to make for himself. The patient should be allowed to make his own deductions at his own pace. In this way the doctor avoids unnecessary antipathy which would otherwise only hinder further cooperation. Furthermore, should the doctor appear too 'clever' his patient may well feel that the doctor is able to read his mind and knows everything even before he himself does. He may either give up the effort of trying to resolve his own problems or withhold information that he assumes the doctor will know through his greater perceptive powers.

It is also especially important during psychoanalysis to refrain from too much interruption. The patient should be allowed time to collect his thoughts and consider carefully what he is saying. A constant barrage of questions by the doctor will distract the patient and often cause him to forget those aspects of his story which he considers important.

The doctor should also exercise restraint in his desire to offer the patient reassurance. In dealing with physical complaints, providing the patient with medical information and thereby resolving unnecessary fears, is an important function of the GP. However, worries based upon emotionally disturbing events should be explored. Mere reassurance in these circumstances will effectively stifle further discussion about them.

The purpose of psychotherapy is to ease the emotional turmoil of the patient. This is achieved by listening to his troubles, providing him with insight about his behaviour and his emotions, and by allowing him to

... should the doctor appear too 'clever' his patient may well feel that the
doctor is able to read his mind and knows everything even before he
himself does.

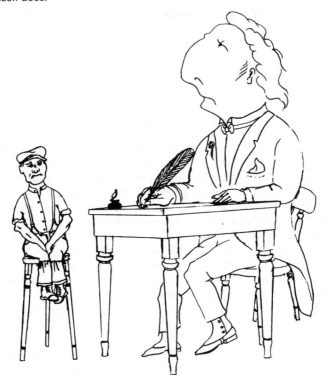

experience those feelings which he has repressed. The results may be
sometimes disappointing even for those with a realistic outlook.
Nevertheless, the relationship that develops between doctor and patient
is honest and worthwhile. Furthermore, psychotherapy provides one
response to the frequent public criticism that general practitioners deal
too dismissively with their patients. It also increases the patient's respect
for his doctor and in many situations helps the patient through some of
his most difficult ordeals.

Chapter 8

Personalities and Problems

'The patient's personality is usually of central importance in all phases of an illness.'
Veikko Tähkä—*The Patient–Doctor Relationship*

Everyone has his own distinctive way of coping with illness. Although the number of symptoms the human body can produce is comparatively few, the variety of ways in which patients may present them is enormous. This is one reason why the problem of diagnosis is far from easy. Understanding the way the patient's personality influences his illness is fundamentally important in general practice. Just as the doctor's personality affects the way in which he conducts his consultations, so the patient's personality will decide the way in which he presents his symptoms. It is necessary for the doctor to be aware of this, for it will enable him to view his patients' illnesses in proper perspective.

The balance of our emotional stability is in a constant state of change. It is modified, particularly in the presence of circumstances which challenge it, and adjusted as we mature. When faced with a particular situation which threatens our emotional stability, we may rise to the occasion and respond in an adult way or, alternatively, as is more frequently the case when we feel unwell and less resilient, we may regress to more childlike forms of behaviour. This fluctuation in our responses has been acknowledged for a long time, but has been described recently in more blatant terms by Berne (1973) in his book *The Games People Play*.

In order to illustrate this point simply I shall confine my attention to a few basic personality types. Though such a restricted focus may be criticized for being too schematic, and, therefore, to some critics will seem unconvincing, I hope it is clear that simple examples help our appreciation of more complex situations.

Most people's personalities, being a mixture of several different personality types, are not clearly circumscribed and do not fit easily into any one single group. Nevertheless, the pattern of their behaviour can be understood from the different facets of their personality. Tähkä (1984) has described this association between personality and illness, and I hope that the following examples which he used, and which I have simplified, will explain how people react differently, so that when, in practice, more complex issues do arise, they will not seem so bewildering.

Excessive Dependence

Quite naturally we all seek comfort and reassurance when we feel ill and, indeed, this is healthy, normal and desirable, if only because it prompts us to seek medical help. There are some people, however, who always remain infantile and immature and who, when ill, become excessively dependent upon others. Similarly a few apparently normal, independent people, when confronted with the uncertainties of ill health, may suddenly regress to this state of childish dependency.

Such patients can be exasperating to deal with. They are excessively self-absorbed, usually demand instant attention, and may even resent the care shown by the doctor to others. Should such individuals develop chronic illness requiring prolonged treatment, they are prone to dependence both upon the drugs they take and upon the doctor. If they have to stay in hospital for a long time, they are also liable to become institutionalized.

The doctor should be aware of such problems and try not to respond with irritation and annoyance. Should he be unable to do this, however, and instead deliberately avoid the patient to minimize the effect of his own feelings, the patient is likely to become even more demanding and frightened, as would an abandoned child. Furthermore, if this situation is allowed to deteriorate, the patient may even begin to develop psychosomatic symptoms and can sometimes become severely depressed.

The doctor should try to remain tolerant of the patient's excessive demands, yet firmly point out that while he understands how the patient must feel, he cannot possibly fulfil all his requests as they are wilfully unrealistic and altogether too demanding. In short, the patient must realize that he cannot always have what he wants.

Excessive Independence

In complete contrast to the above example some people are excessively independent. They consider themselves to be totally self-sufficient and to have no need of help from others. Being so self-reliant, they are unusually tolerant of circumstances which to others would be alarming or unsettling. These 'strong, silent' types meet with much approval for their uncomplaining nature and valiant qualities.

Though they may seem to possess admirable attributes, they do occasionally present serious problems both for themselves and for those who have to cope with them. They delay seeking medical attention until it is often too late and, even when they do, fail to comply with prescribed instructions, considering that they know better than the doctor, and can do just as well without him.

Regrettably, their self-assurance ultimately breaks down as their health progressively deteriorates, and sooner or later they come face to face with their final inability to cope alone. Such confrontation is a watershed. Because of their abhorrence of dependency and their need to push such conclusions to the back of their mind, their eventual realization of failure comes in a sudden flood of anguish, resulting in aggression and hostility and sometimes, because their feelings are directed at themselves, in suicidal depression.

In deciding how best to treat such patients, it is important to encourage them to take a key role in their own management. If suitable alternative forms of treatment are available, the patient should be free to choose between them. Care should be taken to avoid being patronising, or giving the patient the impression that he is being manipulated, both of which would have unfortunate and undesirable consequences. Furthermore, he should not be cossetted, nor be shown excessive sympathy. Any sympathy that is expressed should be directed at acknowledging how difficult it must be for one so independent to cope in the face of such adversity.

Superiority

We all measure our own self-importance and worth by evaluating how well we fulfil our aims and ambitions. To a lesser degree we also rely upon the appraisal of others, although this is more important in childhood. There are some adults, however, with disturbed early relationships, who never rid themselves of their insatiable appetite for praise. Perhaps they protect themselves from acknowledging their real, but suppressed, feelings of insecurity with a delusion of superiority. Their self-satisfaction or narcissism may be based upon any one of a variety of characteristics, such as appearance, knowledge, social position, wealth, or personality.

People with this craving for praise are often admired as they respond so convincingly to a receptive audience, among whom will be many hero-worshippers who have need of someone to idealize. So, although they are conceited and self-absorbed, they may also be ingratiating to those whom they wish to please or impress.

Clearly such people are adversely affected by illness, because it diminishes the effectiveness of their performance and removes them from the environment in which they flourish. Nevertheless, they are quick to turn new situations to their own advantage and, when visiting a doctor, will try to dominate the interview. They may, of course, look upon the doctor as an inferior being, treating him dismissively or patronisingly. They may view the general practitioner especially, as a second rate individual and demand immediate specialist referral, or even bypass the GP altogether. Throughout the interview, the patient will constantly be scrutinizing the doctor for faults and signs of weakness, the seriousness of which he will later magnify in his own mind.

In the face of such arrogance it is difficult for the doctor to behave normally. He will probably feel the insecurity which is being thrust upon him, and in an attempt to reduce his uncertainty, deal with the patient in a hurried way, or comply with his wishes by referring him immediately for a second opinion.

Such management is understandable, but not to be recommended. The doctor will only be respected if he respects himself. He should try to convey some sense of his own worth to the patient by doing a thorough job and by ensuring that the patient is aware of this. Self-assertion by the patient is best matched by self-confidence in the doctor.

Excessive Control

Some people feel secure only when they consider themselves to be totally in control of their environment or the situation in which they find themselves. They are compulsive, and maintain this tight control by resorting to rigid patterns of behaviour which may eventually become ritualized. For example, they may be excessively neat and arrange complicated routines to tidy the home, or keep themselves and their families clean. They may be compulsive in their work and need repeatedly to check not only the quality of their own performance, but often that of their colleagues. Such people have the reputation of being extremely conscientious workers but, because of their anxieties about delegating responsibility, they do experience difficulties when placed in charge of others.

So long as life continues in its usual routine all is well, but many unpredictable circumstances, including illness, will disrupt it, disturbing their peace of mind. The doctor should be aware of how unsettling this can be to such patients and try quickly to re-establish their self-confidence by familiarizing them with the new situation.

Given carefully selected information about the less pessimistic aspects of their illness, these patients will become more relaxed and cooperative, and willing to participate in controlling its progress. However, the doctor should avoid being too candid, as gloomy predictions will be particularly upsetting and merely reinforce their fears that the illness is out of control. Shared care is especially important for compulsive people who, by being involved, will feel reassured in the knowledge that their doctor is treating them thoughtfully, systematically and thoroughly.

Hostility

There are all sorts of reasons why patients become annoyed with their doctors and, as we have seen, anger is sometimes transiently aroused during the consultation. However, some people's personalities have been so damaged, that they are always ready to be aggressive. They are generally unself-critical and tend to perceive that all threats to their well-being, including illness, come from circumstances beyond their control and responsibility. This 'externalization' makes them feel threatened and suspicious of everyone, and clearly damages their personal relationships.

Such patients are extremely provoking and often do their utmost to criticize and unsettle the doctor who, not surprisingly, may rise to the bait and lose his temper. Regrettably however, such a reaction will merely confirm the patient's biased opinions. Because of their need to find fault with everyone but themselves, they are critical of all the institutions which are essentially there to support them, for example social services, employment bureaux, hospitals and general practice, etc.

At work, their employers consider them to be uncooperative and inflexible and, as a consequence, are constantly looking for ways to dismiss them and these individuals for their part, continually find themselves fighting the system to redress the wrongs done to them. They often present to the GP for letters of support or certificates or proof of illness, and the GP often finds himself acquiescing to their demands, against his better judgement. In short, they are thoroughly exasperating people, who are almost impossible to treat satisfactorily.

However, deal with them he must, and the doctor would do well to try to curb his feelings. He should avoid showing too much sympathy as this will only be misinterpreted by the patient as a sign of weakness. Rather, it is better to blunt the thrust of the patient's hostility by remaining detached and conveying to the patient what the doctor considers to be a fair, accurate and honest clinical appraisal of the problem.

Complete breakdown of communication is frequently a problem and when it does occur, it is rarely satisfactorily restored. In these situations it is in the mutual interests of patient and doctor that the patient transfers to another doctor.

Self-reproach and Depression

Physical illness is frequently accompanied by feelings of loss. A reduction in our physical capabilities, and our relative isolation, particularly when confined to bed, no doubt form the basis of this. Quite understandably therefore, we commonly experience an accompanying mood of depression. Provided this is only temporary, we adapt to this change of circumstance, and resign ourselves to some of the meagre compensations that illness brings, namely being cared for, receiving sympathy, freedom from obligations, and the comfort of bed.

In the presence of serious illness, however, where there is no respite in the patient's slow, steady decline, it is not unusual for him to ask himself: 'Why me? What have I done to deserve this?' Self-pity is translated into self-reproach. Suffering is often interpreted as a form of punishment arising from feelings of guilt.

One of the problems a doctor has to face when dealing with people who are depressed, is assessing the possible risk of suicide. Very often, those who are at risk will readily acknowledge it, but surprise suicides do occur, and it can be a real worry for the doctor trying to identify them.

Signs of emotional detachment may often mislead the inexperienced doctor to conclude that the patient is not so seriously depressed, but this is a dangerous paradox. The absence of feeling for others, especially those negative feelings of anger and reproach, may signify that all the patient's hatred is involuted or directed towards himself. Because of his detachment the patient will fail to make emotional appeals for help and so conceal the serious risk of suicide (Tähkä, 1984).

Caution is also required in treating those with feelings of guilt and reproach. It is better not to express too much sympathy for these patients, as they will probably feel unworthy of it, which will enhance their guilt. Tähkä suggests that they are best treated by adopting a regimen which is both firm and caring. He maintains that this makes the patient feel confident in his treatment and yet still allows him to grumble against authority. It gives him the necessary outlet for the reproach which would otherwise be unleashed against himself.

Self-pity

Although self-pity is usually a passing mood that we all experience from time to time, there are some people whose mental stability greatly depends on it. For them self-pity is a permanent reaction to their hostility.

Such people are martyrs and unconsciously seek out situations which will allow them to feel sorry for themselves. They are often wilfully self-effacing and may go to extraordinary lengths to put themselves out for the benefit of others, in order to show how self-sacrificing they are. Though they may not always grumble directly, they often drop broad hints in conversation about how ill-treated they consider themselves to be. Together with this unconscious search for situations which will be to their disadvantage, they also tend to distort their memory of past events, recounting them in a way which will show how unfortunate they have been.

Paradoxically, sympathy is not really what they want. In spite of drawing attention to their sufferings, they are actually expressing their need for humiliation. When first confronted with such people, the natural reaction is to feel sorry for them, but very quickly sympathy is replaced by irritation. Yet again, this demonstrates how effective they are at turning situations around to increase their self-pity and humiliation.

When dealing with such a patient, the doctor should restrain himself from too much consolation or encouraging the patient into better health by saying how much better he is looking. This will merely frustrate the patient's basic need. Showing reasonable sympathy is enough and will demonstrate to the patient that the doctor has understood how hard it must be to suffer so.

However, it is in the nature of the patient's personality to find faults, and sooner or later he will want to feel that the doctor has mismanaged or neglected him. Provided that the doctor is willing to tolerate this situation, it will reasonably suit the patient. If the doctor can curtail his need to prove to the patient how competent he is and how good are his intentions, he will be doing what the patient requires (Balint, 1964). Psychotherapy is ineffective and undesirable for such people as self-pity is often their only alternative substitute for depression.

Withdrawal

Physical illness is usually associated with a certain degree of withdrawal. This is entirely healthy and allows the person to concentrate upon himself, his illness and his recovery. However, there are some people with 'schizoid' personalities who are permanently withdrawn. They are loners and illness makes them more so.

Far from being insensitive, they seek isolation to remove the fearful intrusion that close relationships involve. Withdrawal is for them a protective mechanism and should not be threatened, nor should they be actively encouraged to make friendships or enter into the social activities of others. Rather they should be treated courteously and with a certain reserve and detachment, yet at the same time allowing them the opportunity to make the first move towards better contact, should they wish.

Infatuation and Eroticism

Patients with hysterical personalities frequently have fantasies which, in the presence of severe emotional disturbance, may lead to complex delusions. Such fantasies are often a substitute for real fulfilment, so dissatisfaction with a close personal relationship can provide the need in such a patient to find imaginery satisfaction elsewhere. A sympathetic doctor is an obvious point of focus.

Such patients will often go to considerable efforts to make themselves attractive to the doctor, and may eventually, either by gesture or declaration, reveal their feelings for him/her. When so confronted, it is inappropriate to appear prudish or moralistic. The doctor should refrain from reacting impulsively, as though in imminent danger of being summoned before a disciplinary tribunal but, on the other hand, ought to be careful and avoid fuelling the patient's fantasies.

It is preferable to maintain a spontaneous and friendly approach towards the patient, while firmly preserving a professional role. The doctor should discuss the patient's feelings tactfully, so as not to damage the patient's self-respect, and yet at the same time provide a sound factual basis to their relationship. This enables the patient to distinguish between reality and fantasy.

In some instances the patient's emotional stability will be so disturbed that fantasies give way to delusions and, despite the doctor's repeated assurances to the contrary, the patient is convinced that the feelings of love are reciprocated. Such patients should probably be referred to a psychiatrist of the same sex, if this is possible.

Chapter 9

Character Unfolding:
The Doctor's Personality

'The risk would remain, even with close knowledge of Lydgate's character; for character too is a process and an unfolding. The man was still in the making, as much as the Middlemarch doctor and immortal discoverer, and there were both virtues and faults capable of shrinking or expanding.'

George Eliot—*Middlemarch*

So far, we have discussed problems which arise from the patient's personality, but it is important to realize that difficulties may also result from the doctor's personality and his reaction to the patient. The doctor should recognize this and be aware of his own personality traits, otherwise he will have no sense of perspective with which to view his relationship with his patients.

Michael O'Donnell, family doctor and celebrated broadcaster and journalist is very well aware of this. With characteristic humour he wrote about many such examples in his book *Doctor! Doctor!—An Insider's Guide to the Games Doctors Play* (1986).

For example a doctor who is excessively independent and stoical may well consider that his patients ought to behave similarly. When confronted by a patient who is prone to self-pity, the GP will be inclined to dismiss him as pathetic and undeserving of his care and attention. While such feelings may be understandable, they are not at all appropriate and should not be expressed. Furthermore, since emotions may be inadvertently conveyed by gesture or inference, the doctor should take particular care to control them. He may only do this successfully if he is fully aware of their presence and origin, and can appreciate their destructive influence.

Somewhat in contrast to this, the doctor who is inclined to feel sorry for himself will also pose problems. He may well make a martyr of himself by insisting upon visiting every patient who makes a request for advice. He may also make repeat home visits unnecessarily, often to demonstrate how heavy is his own work load compared with that of his partners who, he thinks consequently, are not doing their share of the practice work. Such a long-suffering doctor is as tiresome to himself as he is to his colleagues and, as well as generating unnecessary work, encourages his patients to become unduly dependent upon him.

Superiority is another problem. Arrogance in a doctor always distances him from his patients. Previously we have seen how, in the past, doctors may have relied for their success upon their authority and the relative complicity of their patients. When patients are ignorant, this may be successful, but in an increasingly informed society, it is misplaced and very often damaging. Such doctors will rarely seem sympathetic, and their authority is a poor substitute for imaginative concern when dealing with patients who are emotionally upset.

To illustrate some of these problems more fully, I shall pay greater attention to a few personality types, just as I have done with the patient. In an effort to simplify the dynamics, I have focused upon certain specific characteristics. It is important to realize, however, that in reality we are all a blend of many types, and each one is merely a facet upon which our world is reflected.

The true picture that we project is a kaleidoscope of tones, shapes and colours each reacting with the other in an ever changing spectrum.

For character too is a process and an unfolding.
George Eliot—*Middlemarch*

The Controlling Doctor

The number of patients that a GP can successfully manage will vary appreciably, and depends not only upon his capacity for work, but also on his personality. It will very much determine his style of consultation, and his style will determine it.

In 1954 Lord Taylor, probably in response to the burden imposed upon GPs after the flood gates of the new NHS had been opened in 1948, said: 'The doctor with the heavy work-load will do well to avoid all unnecessary talk with his patients. It is a high clinical skill to make patients express themselves adequately in the shortest possible time. The primary purpose of contact between patient and doctor, namely the making of the correct medical diagnosis and the application of the right treatment, must never be allowed to get lost in a flood of verbosity on either side.'

Faced with such heavy demands, where safety and the elimination of distraction are paramount, control becomes a necessity. Nowadays, however, the demands have changed, as too have patients' expectations. Patient autonomy is now more widely accepted, whilst the doctor's exclusive authority less tolerated.

So the GP who feels that his prime duty is to heal physical illness, and who as a result of this, believes that his time is being wasted with trivia when confronted with worries that he considers have no medical foundation, is likely to suffer much dissatisfaction.

This will be reflected in his manner. At best he may try to restrict the patient's story to that which is organic and dismiss the rest as irrelevant and hypochondriacal, or worse he may become irritated, unsympathetic, curt and even abrasive. He may see many of his patients as time wasters, and will try to limit the time they waste. He will strive to tighten his control upon the consultation and will probably take satisfaction from being a good time keeper. He will no doubt be able to deal swiftly with his patients, keeping to remarkably consistent appointment schedules.

As his technique has its distant origins in that which he learned at Medical School, he may delude himself into thinking that his consultations are efficient and safe. They are neither. So much may be missed and there is too little time to form a considered opinion. There is also so much distortion from his attempts to extract a clear story, when in reality it may be anything but. Patients may also withhold important information when confronted with an abrupt manner or even fabricate a story when rushed into responding to difficult questions.

In such instances the patient may leave bemused at what went on, or even angry with themselves and the doctor.

'When I got there and sat down, I didn't dare tell him .... In fact I told him a whole string of lies' (a patient's comment after the consultation—Stimson and Webb, 1975).

A controlling doctor will attract to himself those patients who enjoy being controlled and who prefer punctuality to other considerations, or can precis their thoughts for a quick encounter. His patients will learn to marshall their ideas well beforehand and will expect a predictable outcome. In short the consultation is contained and finite, but little else. Furthermore his patients, when visiting other partners with a more open approach, may well feel irritated at being kept waiting longer than usual for their appointment, and unsettled by a less directed consultation. They may also feel alarmed or affronted by questions which for them represent intrusions into privacy.

Despite their enviable habit of disciplined timekeeping, controlling doctors seldom learn the true value of listening. Their consultations are so tightly reined and selective, that there is neither the time nor the latitude for imaginative thought. For them the consultation becomes locked into a regime of question, answer, and reflex response. Much of what the patient presents will be filtered and restrained, and most of the content reduced to trivialities. 'The doctor spoke dispassionately, almost brutally, with the relish men of science sometimes have for limiting themselves to inessentials, for pruning back their work to the point of sterility' (Evelyn Waugh—*Brideshead Revisited*).

As there is no room for development, the opportunity to learn about people and behaviour, the very essence of general practice, will be lost. The assessment of his patients' personalities and their emotional problems by such a doctor will be, for the most part, facile and sometimes breathtakingly wide of the mark. Such doctors often become bored and disillusioned with their work, and the technique of their consultation arrested in its early development.

Probably in the past many GPs were like this, accounting for the regrettable findings of Ann Cartwright's surveys between 1964 and 1981. Whilst it is possible for a doctor to learn much about life through the vast number of consultations conducted throughout his professional career, it is equally possible for him to learn very little.

Such a doctor may feel entirely self-satisfied and consider himself to be efficient, yet due largely to his brittle attitude and unapproachability he is unaware of so many of his omissions, which are often left to be fielded by his partners. Furthermore in his dealings with them, he is sure-footed in offering his own opinions and so unreceptive to theirs, that there is seldom common ground for compromise. Grievances against him will never be adequately aired in practice meetings, and resentments against him will surface from time to time throughout his working life.

The Excessively Sympathetic Doctor

Sympathy is an important requirement for any GP, but it should not be dispensed without restraint. Unfortunately there are some doctors who are excessively sympathetic, and need to feel liked whatever the cost. These doctors will spend inordinate amounts of time with their patients, who, for the most part, will be grateful and appreciative. Their consultations will be open ended, and their time keeping usually relaxed. Their style is often patient-led but not always so, and problems are conscientiously and sometimes exhaustively investigated, sometimes unnecessarily so. They will be highly praised by many of their patients who like to demonstrate their appreciation at Christmas time.

Unfortunately, because such doctors are not always disciplined and selective in their offers of sympathy, they attract a disproportionate number of hypochondriacs. In one respect, this may be seen as a benefit for other partners in the practice, who may discover their own hypochondriacal patients drifting across to the doctor they prefer but there are disadvantages. Because many of these patients' problems are insoluble, and take up so much fruitless time for inquiry, investigation, follow-up and reinvestigation, such doctors are booked up well in advance. Vacant appointments are not sufficiently available for their other patients, who inevitably drift in the opposite direction to be picked up by the other partners. This may cause some exasperation within the practice, especially among those who feel that the exorbitant demands of hypochondriacs should not be pandered to, particularly at the expense of sick patients.

Furthermore, in providing so much time for these patients, the doctor reinforces their dependency upon him, and they never learn to be independent and reassure themselves. Whenever they get the slightest problem, they rush off back to the doctor. This reinforcing behaviour often affects younger members of the patient's family inculcating further hypochondriacal patterns of behaviour in them.

Hypochondriasis is one of the most difficult of all the common conditions with which a GP has to deal. The aim of management should be to break the cycle of problem and anxiety. The usual repeated visits to the doctor offer only temporary respite, and is no lasting solution.

A better alternative is to persuade the patient to acknowledge his condition and search for its cause. Of course, this is only likely to be achieved, provided the doctor shows no disparagement. The term 'hypochondriac' carries with it such a stigma, that the mere mention of the name to some patients can cause immense indignation.

The origins of hypochondria normally arise from learnt responses in childhood, namely from the witnessing of parental hypochondriacal behaviour by their children. These families will have several members, spanning several generations, with numerous complaints and thick medical records. Yet they live to a ripe old age. Occasionally, however, hypochondriasis might arise as a singular event, for example in a child who suddenly becomes seriously ill, destroying its peace of mind and its previously held assumptions to a right to good health. Then without any adequate explanation to the child, it is suddenly plucked from the security of home and rushed to hospital for a whole catalogue of nasty events. Such medical miscommunication proclaims to the child that the comfort of everyday life can, without warning, be suddenly shattered. How is it to know in future that a trivial sore throat or innocuous stomach-ache won't be the herald of an un-predictably dangerous condition? Suddenly life becomes very uncertain and frightening.

Whatever the cause of their hypochondriasis, patients need a doctor whom they can trust. Not surprisingly, the excessively sympathetic doctor is the one doctor whom they will trust, and he is best placed to achieve a lasting cure, but unless he makes more selective and creative use of his sympathy he is unlikely to achieve it. However, once the patient has realized the true source of his condition, he may mature to independence and self-assurance (*Hypochondria: Woeful Imaginings.* Susan Baur (1988).).

The Excessively Conscientious Doctor

For most who enter general practice, the overriding attraction is the sheer variety of conditions with which patients present. Not for them the endless repetition of cases seen in outpatients where the diagnosis has often already been made.

For a few, however, this panoply of illness is unsettling. These GPs are never reconciled to the aphorism often fondly quoted by older members of their profession: 'You just never know what next will walk in through that door.'

For them it is a fear rather than a fascination, and one that they can contain only with exhaustive history taking, compulsive systems review, and endless investigation. It is as though they are locked into the role of new houseman, unable to come to any firm conclusions and with the prospect of the most vague symptom, pointing to a possible medical horror.

With increasing litigation, the amazing variety of general practice can become a nightmare. For them restricting the consultation to a brief encounter is a minefield of worry. Consequently they toil over every concern, leaving nothing to chance, each slight symptom being treated with monumental thoroughness, warranting endless investigation and follow-up.

Because the prevailing attitude of the doctor is one of caution, his patients come to expect full investigation for the most trivial of symptoms. Though they may not all be hypochondriacal, they can become increasingly difficult to reassure without such tests. For doctors taking over the care of such patients, difficulty arises in trying to return to a more acceptable level of management. A few patients may even become hypochondriacal as a result of such scrupulous care. After inherited family behaviour, medical mismanagement is the second commonest factor in the development of this condition (Susan Baur—*Hypochondria: Woeful Imaginings.*).

This cycle of over-investigation induces dependency and is good for neither patient nor doctor, although his colleagues may be occasionally beneficially reassured by asking him to see one of their bewildering problems on the basis that if he can't sort it out no one can.

Though his notes may be exhaustively long, they lead often to inconclusive and concomitantly long differential diagnoses. Far from being an *aide memoire* they rapidly become a mass of unmanageable information. Sadly because there is so much information acquired, important diagnoses that might otherwise have been obvious, can be missed.

Often the scrupulous doctor gets exasperated with himself at failing to discover that tantalizingly elusive diagnosis, and sometimes with his partners for failing to properly look after his patients in his absence. Some such GPs are aware of their meticulousness but can do little to rid themselves of it, whilst others feel justified with their actions and conclude that general practice does not deserve them.

Eventually many suffer from professional 'burn out', and a few resign themselves to the fact they are unsuited to life as a GP, because it holds too many uncertainties.

The Busy Doctor

Because doctors are paid according to the size of their list, many accept more patients than they can comfortably manage. Some may be motivated by money, but others by other considerations. It may gratify them to know that they have more patients than their colleagues. It enhances their feeling of self-worth, and helps erase any criticism they may imagine from their partners that they are not pulling their weight: for them one of the worst faults.

They may have difficulty in turning patients away, deluding themselves that, no matter what, they can cope. Such doctors will be extremely busy, and the foundation of their work ethic is their refusal to turn work away: their difficulty in saying 'no'.

Sometimes, for self-gratification or in order to reinforce their self-importance, they boast their busy schedule to colleagues, staff and patients. In short their self-esteem is dependent upon the amount they do. The busier they are, the more important they feel.

They invariably have other commitments outside the practice, and they find themselves dashing here, there and everywhere under constant pressure of time. They are the busiest of doctors, but much of their tribulation is of their own making.

In order to cope with this exhausting schedule, they have frequently to cut corners, and develop the nack of diagnosis from intuitive hunches. They are often rapid fire information gatherers, but not always so, and can display a range of consultation techniques. They may change tack in styles and are very adept at speeding up in the latter consultations of a busy surgery, to recover from the inevitable delays and interruptions that are the daily diet of the busy GP.

Though they accept the adverse consequences of telephone interruptions, such doctors may make no attempt to curtail them, as this would be an admission to themselves of their failure to be able to cope. These all add to the delay, and the doctor then responds with a subsequent shift in emphasis to a much more controlling, doctor-centred style.

In speeding up, the GP may be tempted to jump in with premature questions, without listening to the whole of the patient's response, or, when faced with a hesitant patient, even to complete his answers for him. Vital information may be lost, and the whole direction of the consultation, occasionally, radically shifted. Explanations to the patient may be hurried or even omitted, and the patient denied the opportunity of grasping the doctor's message. The patient may leave the surgery with only a vague notion of what was said, or even a false idea of the instructions given.

In such instances, the therapeutic information will be left to the pharmacist and not surprisingly confusion and mistakes do arise. Because the busy doctor may have dashed off to other outside appointments, the misunderstanding may have to be resolved by his partners, who can only wonder and guess, particularly if, in his haste, the busy GP has failed to keep adequate notes.

Such doctors may never have time to reflect upon what they do, and so never realize that the root cause of their harassment is themselves. They may, and frequently do, feel resentful that they are doing the lion's share of the work. This feeling is often mirrored in the busy doctor's spouse who feels neglected and annoyed often with the partners for allowing this to happen.

Whilst they both feel that the other partners in the practice should take on more of the work, the workalcoholic GP would do well to consider doing less himself.

Token Empathy: The 'I've had that' Doctor

Sympathy and empathy are expressions of feeling which when shared may provide immense therapeutic benefit. Every day, however, doctors are presented with problems that may evoke such sentiments, and their expressions of sympathy can become routine without much real feeling, seeming insincere or even disingenuous.

The patient may feel patronized, teased or even belittled, especially if he interprets the gesture of feigned sympathy on the doctor's face as a smile of indifference or a smirk.

A not infrequent habit that some doctors have, and which commonly causes irritation, is to claim to have had the same illness with which the patient is presenting. This will probably be done in a cheery, slightly dismissive way in a misguided attempt to appease the patient's worries. It is as though the GP were saying, 'Oh! I've had that. It is nothing to worry about. You'll get over it, just like I did.'

Some patients may be reassured, but others will not, the outcome depending largely on the doctor's manner and his relationship with the patient. A few will find it irritating, although it may not have been intended to be an uncaring remark. It is, therefore, better avoided or limited to a few special occasions.

If the doctor does have a genuine personal experience of the condition or investigation, empathy can be better expressed through his greater understanding and awareness of the patient's plight, and by gently detailing those areas of particular difficulty, with an emphasis on reassurance. However, there may be a few occasions when it can be helpful to admit to personal experience. If he does so when his habit is usually one of restraint, his expression of empathy is more likely to be genuine and not a mere token.

The Jolly Doctor and the Joker

A sense of humour is generally considered to be an essential quality for a GP, making him resilient to the stresses and emotional buffeting that face him every day. Transference of feeling between patient and doctor is a commonly shared experience. A cheerful doctor often makes his patients feel better merely with his presence, whilst he himself avoids being made depressed by his patients, because he is so bouyant. Such a doctor is held in much affection by his patients, who will overlook many of his professional shortcomings. In fact, he is often so loved by his patients that, in times of great crisis, they will see no one else, preferring to wait until he is available rather than see one of his partners. This is particularly the case at times of personal tragedy. It is as though the doctor had been adopted by the family as the favourite uncle to whom all woes must be told.

He is likely to be extrovert and big hearted as well as sympathetic and down to earth. However, he may not necessarily be analytical or self-critical, and many of his responses are born of innate feeling and gut reactions. So confident is he of his responses, that when he does draw a false conclusion, he may be unaware of it and may dismiss out of hand contrary propositions to correct his view point.

His success as a healer will be based upon his sympathy and his benevolent humour, and most of his patients will leave his surgery with a lighter heart than when they entered.

In marked contrast, however, there are some doctors who regularly use humour as a form of control, making jokey, tactless remarks to the patient at his or her expense. Sometimes his remarks are oblique and snide, at other times direct. Some patients will be affronted, others perplexed, and left wondering if they have interpreted the inference correctly. Either way when directed at emotionally vulnerable patients, these remarks can be very hurtful.

Some patients will enjoy the banter and will refer to their doctor as a bit of a card, but many will dislike him, while his partners will have to shoulder much of his work, as patients ultimately drift away from him.

Consultation with the joking doctor are predictably superficial and dismissive, and conclusions facile, often being fabricated to fit the humour rather than the patient's diagnosis. The interface of the interview is unyielding and confrontational, and the time provided barely adequate. This is one of the unacceptable faces of personality, as much of the control is achieved at the patient's expense.

The Unacceptable Face of Personality

No matter how rigorous the selection of medical students becomes, there will always be doctors whose character develops in unacceptable ways. It is the duty of all professions to police their members, and doctors who commit serious breaches of conduct will find themselves temporarily suspended or struck off the register.

Grave misconduct within the consultation can have profoundly damaging consequences, not only to the patient and his relatives, but also, by reflection, on the rest of the medical profession.

Alcohol, drug and sexual abuse are some of the most frequent examples. A common association between these three is a failure by the doctor to accept that his habit is out of control, or that it is damaging himself and his patients. Offenders frequently allow themselves a little latitude in interpreting their code of ethics which they consider too rigid. They maintain that to do so is merely human, and moroever only liberal and more relaxed. They also delude themselves with the notion that their frequent habit is not yet an addiction, and is well within their command. The effect of drugs and alcohol does much to foster this deception, and paradoxically makes them feel in better control, an important consideration for them with the concurrent stress that is commonly present in their lives.

In the case of sexual misconduct the doctor, who is more often than not male, may well be aided by the patient who occasionally does encourage it. In this, however, the guilty doctor fails to realize that the patient's compliance is invariably a response to her own domestic and emotional situation, which needs to be treated rather than taken advantage of.

Much sexual abuse by doctors is nothing more than physical self-gratification, but some doctors, as part of their need to be liked and admired, deliberately seek out immature and emotionally vulnerable patients of the opposite gender, ostensibily to offer them counselling. The women the doctor selects are emotionally frustrated, yearning for a fulfilling sexual partnership. The intense focus of psychotherapy provides the setting, and before long both doctor and patient believe they are in love with each other.

This may well be true of the patient, though she is often unaware that she is responding to seriously misleading cues, but for the doctor it is nothing more than emotional manipulation for his own distorted needs. Such a doctor rarely restricts himself to one such patient, and may have several. So genuine may his intentions seem, that his susceptible victims can scarcely see through his deception, even when he is eventually brought to book at a disciplinary hearing, and they have to appear as witnesses.

Alcohol abuse and drugs of addiction both cause serious disturbances of personality. Not only do they adversely affect performance, but they also alter character. Perhaps there was a time when patients were tolerant of such lapses, but the dangers of such behaviour are now so well known, that it is totally unacceptable. The GP addict has such easy access to the source of his habit, that he should not be allowed to continue within this branch of the profession. Should he do so, he is a constant danger to himself, his partners and his patients, as well as other road users when he is on his rounds.

His behaviour may be so disinhibited that he goes beyond the bounds of propriety, both during his consultation and when examining the patient. His skill, reasoning, conclusions and treatment may all be seriously impaired, and his disturbed behaviour presents his partners with major problems.

It would be possible to continue with many more examples, but my purpose in providing these few is simply to provide an awareness of how personality affects outcome, and how little heed is generally paid towards this in medical education. The examples I have selected are, of course, stylized. In reality, our own true characters are a blend of several such examples. I have intentionally focused on specific empirical types, in order to ease understanding. No doubt you may recognize different facts of yourself in some of the categories I have described. The emphasis of this chapter is not to discourage variety, but to make you aware of it, to accept it, improve on its benefits both to you and the patients, minimize its deficiencies and eradicate any harm.

So marked is this effect of personality upon the consultation that it is probable that the same patient with the same presenting complaint be accorded a thorough and lengthy deliberation from one doctor, and yet from another be shown the door in almost no time at all. Furthermore, such extremes of variation can be true for the same patient and the same GP but for different circumstances, dependent upon the doctor's mood and the extent to which he responds to pressure of time and harassment.

Scarce wonder then, that we all, even the most conscientious, are capable, at one time or another, of indifferent and even bad practice.

So, just from these few brief examples, we can see that the interplay of personalities between doctor and patient is extremely varied and adds to the interest and complexity of their relationship. Because of the great diversity of problems and personalities in general practice, it is inappropriate to promote any one single consultation style or technique. Flexibility is an enormous asset for the doctor, but should he not possess it or be unable to develop it, he must be true to himself and maintain the style which best suits him, and which ultimately will be the most satisfactory compromise for his patients.

Whatever style he adopts, however, the GP should avoid complacency and maintain his self-critical faculties, be vigilant about his mistakes, and be prepared to review his performance regularly throughout his professional life.

Chapter 10

The Illusion of Objectivity:
The Doctor–Patient Relationship

'The sole tool that we bring to the task of understanding others is our own personality. The cues we receive from the outside must be processed through the perceptual equipment that is "us"—through lenses of our own background and expectations. If we are to be successful in assessing the meaning of cues that impinge on us, we must become aware of the distortions that may be introduced by our "built-in" perceptual equipment.'
Massarik F. and Wechsler I. R. – *Empathy Revisited*

The categorization of a person's character is neither fixed nor rigidly determined, even if it were possible to take account of every facet. It is always relative, and also variable. Character is a process rather than a state. Moreover our perception of character, namely how we think of ourselves and how we think of others, is also relative and variable.

We never see ourselves in isolation, merely in relation to one another, both past and present. Not only do relationships affect character and how we behave, but they also determine how we interpret and assess it. In short, personality is a function of social intercourse, constructed and determined by language.

To simplify the theory, I hope the following example will help. A sixth form student might be confident among his peers at school, and see himself as an intellectual superior, sure in the knowledge that he is cleverer than the rest. Once he goes to University, however, he could feel considerably less secure, and might even experience strongly negative feelings towards himself and his previously held self-assurance. His self-awareness is strongly influenced by his environment, and his personality also is shaped by it.

This is true for all aspects of character, rather in the way that colour is intensified or muted by whatever other colour is placed next to it, and the light which illuminates it.

'Kenneth Gergen, social psychologist, set out to show how peoples' self-esteem and their self-concept changed in sheer reaction to the kinds of people they found themselves among, and changed even more in response to the positive or negative remarks that people made to them. Even if they were asked to play a particular public role in a group, their self-image often changed in a fashion to be congruent with that role. Indeed, in the presence of others who were older or seen to be more powerful than they were, people would report on "self" in a quite different and diminishing way from their manner of seeing themselves when in the presence of younger or less-esteemed people'.

John Woodall (1996)

To illustrate this more fully using the analogy of colour, I have drawn a personality wheel, rather like a colour wheel (Fig. 10.1). This is used only as a way of illustrating how facets of character may influence each other. I do not suggest that it would be used to categorize personality, which, in the event, would be facile.

On the empirical basis that opposites attract, I have put opposing character traits diametrically opposite each other, where they can be considered like complementary colours. Similarly, character traits placed side by side on the wheel, have a bias towards each other. Though this is artifically contrived, it may serve to illustrate a useful point.

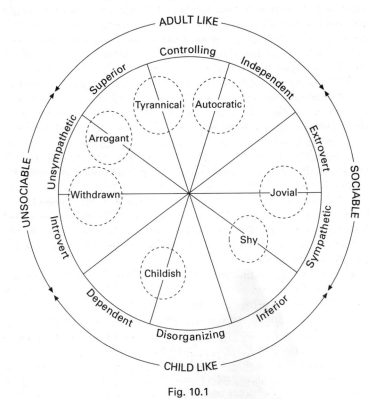

Fig. 10.1

For example, when someone who is superior and controlling, namely a tyrannical type is confronted by an independent, controlling type who is autocratic, there is likely to be a clash of personalities. How each person sees himself is decided by how either of them interprets the outcome of this clash.

In contrast, when a controller is faced with someone who is compliant and dependent, and feels secure in being organized, the outcome is likely to be quite different. Moreover the feelings the controller will have about himself in such a situation are likely to be in marked contrast with how he would have felt when faced with the previously mentioned conflict.

These reactions are just as true for the relationship between patient and doctor as for any other. Perhaps we should be impressed by how similar are our conclusions about patients than by how different they are, but then, perhaps not? As our characters unfold, they are shaped by the professional discipline we have adopted, and by our colleagues within the profession.

Nevertheless such influences do have a profound effect on our relations with patients, and our conclusions about them, and our management of their illnesses. To draw any valid or useful deduction, therefore, we must be aware of our own influence upon the patient, and of the patient's influence on us, either intensifying or neutralizing, complementing or conflicting.

This already difficult situation is further complicated by factors about which we are unaware. In reaching any conclusion, one is only ever aware of that which is conscious. There is a whole world of influence, played by both parties, from their subconscious. This leaves us in a very uncertain world where conclusions can never be anything but circumspect. But this is true also of colour, and it has not prevented the colourists from making many intriguing observations about it.

For doctors who prefer the clear focus of simple truths, general practice will be fraught with exasperation and anxiety. Only those who find such uncertainty acceptable, and even intriguing, will feel at home. Aristotle once said 'There is no such thing as absolute certainty, only the certainty which befits the subject.'

For general practice this certainty is very uncertain indeed. In fact, the art of general practice has been described as the art of managing uncertainty. The reaction between the doctor's and the patient's character, one with another, is one of the foundations of healing. It accounts for the placebo effect, and the power of all healers from time immemorial, even when the treatment itself was ineffective or harmful.

To put this theory into a practical setting, I shall choose for my example the 'overanxious mother'. This pejorative label used to be more frequently seen in GP notes and hospital letters than it is now, largely I suspect, because patients have been entitled since 1991 to look at their medical records.

The term 'overanxious' immediately presupposes that there is an acceptable level of anxiety beyond which it becomes abnormal. Whilst there may be some truth in this, the boundary between a normal anxious reaction and an abnormal one is vague, and will depend above all else upon the cause. To say that someone is anxious or overanxious is neither helpful nor especially informative, and probably reveals more of the doctor's character than the patient's.

If a mother seems anxious, it is essential to establish why. She is likely to be naturally worried by her sick child. She could have reached an alarming conclusion about her child's ailment. She may have previously experienced a similar situation that was serious. She could have a phobia about doctors. More specifically, she could feel intimidated and anxious by the doctor who is now examining her sick child. She might be well informed and equally imaginative, and discover during the consultation that the doctor seems alarmingly ignorant. The possibilities go on.

These, however, are multiplied into even greater permutations by those variables particular to the doctor, who may simply have forgotten, or never have known, how worrying it is to be the parent of a sick child. He may habitually dismiss most of his patients as anxious. He may be anxious himself and try to assuage his own fears by dismissing those of others. He may feel out of his depth, especially if confronted with a patient who knows more than he on the subject. In an attempt to conceal his ignorance he may try to fill the vacuum in his knowledge with a confusing and meaningless circumlocution, forever skirting round the subject, never achieving clarity and generating more worry and exasperation in the patient. He may be dismissive of the condition, recognizing that it is trivial, yet have neither the patience nor the imagination to realise that the mother's fear results from her own thoughts and ideas rather than his. Once again the possibilities are numerous.

To form any worthwhile conclusion and minimize uncertainty, the doctor must have a clear understanding and respect for the mother's worry and have sufficient self-awareness to acknowledge his own role, if any, in this.

Only through this awareness of himself and his patients, and their mutual interplay of character, will the GP be really successful and reap the full rewards from his work. This, however, will not be achieved overnight. It takes considerable time to begin to know patients well enough, but the general practitioner is of all doctors one of the best placed in the profession to achieve this task. As Aristotle said 'For the achievement of any work regarded as an end there must be a prior exercise of many energies or acquired facilities of a secondary order, demanding patience.'

Chapter 11

Similes, Metaphors and Simple Explanations

' ... the doctor himself may be the most potent drug which he prescribes. However, this particular prescription takes a great deal longer in the writing.'
F. Fitton and H. W. K. Acheson—*Doctor/Patient Relationship*

'He didn't tell me anything. Just gave me the prescription.'
Quote from a dissatisfied patient taken from F. Fitton and H. W. K. Acheson—*Doctor/Patient Relationship*

General practitioners frequently fail to provide patients with adequate explanations for their symptoms (Byrne and Long, 1976; Cartwright and Anderson, 1981; Tuckett, 1982). In fact so frequent is this failure, that it is difficult to avoid making the conclusion that it is more by intention than by chance. Doctors who habitually fail to offer explanations do so to maintain authority over their patients. Dr John Pickles unashamedly had this approach and used to boast: 'If they ask me what's wrong with them, I say to them, that's my business. Do as I tell you and take your medicine and you'll get better.'

Perhaps in the past the success of a doctor was based upon his authority and the comparative ignorance of his patients, but today this seems unacceptable. Patients are more knowledgeable and not inclined to be treated dismissively. Attempts by doctors to do so cause mistrust and dissatisfaction, which is scarcely a satisfactory start to treatment. The doctor himself may be the best placebo, yet if he wastes the opportunity, his treatment is much less likely to be effective.

We have already discussed the importance of being aware of patients' own ideas about their symptoms and of dealing with them in a sympathetic way. Only by doing so will reassurance have any value.

The way to achieve this is first to acknowledge to the patient that the sense he makes of his illness is quite understandable. Then, if his theories are valid, those too must be acknowledged. If they are not, the doctor should say so, giving his reasons clearly and simply, and without being patronizing or appearing too clever. Some of the patient's ideas may be based upon false medical information or inaccurate conclusions, which must be corrected. The doctor needs to be tactful to avoid irritating the patient, for it is important to sustain his attention and cooperation throughout to prevent further misunderstanding.

For most consultations the patient's problem is straightforward and requires little explanation. Nevertheless, even for simple requests such as a prescription for a sore throat, it is certainly worthwhile discussing the limitations of treatment. So often patients who initially want a prescription, eventually choose not to have one when told the relevant information. It is unlikely that the patient will be satisfied with a mere bald refusal to his request. He may accept that the doctor knows more about it, but he will still feel peeved, unless he understands why a prescription is unnecessary.

Diagnoses and Labels

Doctors have a professional obligation to make the most accurate diagnosis they reasonably can. Not only is this intellectually rewarding for themselves, but it is reassuring for patients. Though naturally preferring to be told they are well, patients may be more relieved to be given a diagnosis than offered bland and meaningless reassurance. Not surprisingly, they feel that once their condition is recognized and no longer a mystery, there is probably a well-tried form of treatment for it, and if not, they at least have the consolation of knowing that there are others with the same problem. It also provides them with official confirmation that their symptoms are acknowledged to be genuine and not considered to be imaginary or put on, a worry that is common to almost everyone who becomes unwell.

Especially when the prognosis is good and when the doctor is sure of his diagnosis, it is important to tell the patient what this is, and not to withhold it. Sometimes it may be helpful to write it down and hand it to the patient, as this avoids the sort of misunderstandings which may arise from complicated medical jargon, and which, as we have seen in a previous chapter, may lead to considerable and unnecessary anguish.

Such diagnostic labels often give much relief and, at the same time, generate confidence. Arnold Bloom stresses the importance of this in helping to provide reassurance. However, caution is needed if the prognosis is poor, or when the problem is emotional. Terms such as hypochondriasis, neurosis, obsessionalism and so forth are so commonly misapplied by the public, and used in a pejorative sense, that patients so labelled may understandably feel indignant, as it then becomes difficult for them to claim, especially to their friends and relations, that their suffering is real. In these circumstances, if a diagnosis is offered, it is important to use wording which still allows the patient to retain his self-respect and dignity.

However some would argue that the emotional problems most frequently seen in general practice are not easily categorized or given

Explanations are worthless unless they are understood, so it is important to use simple and clear language without unnecessary jargon.

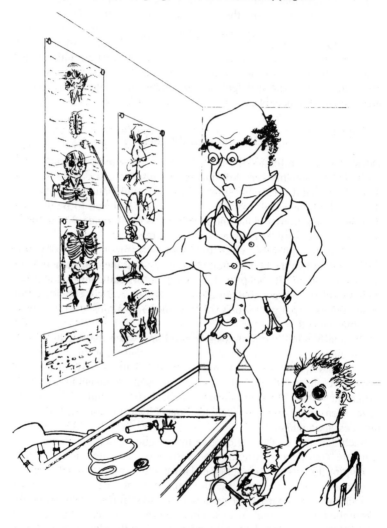

diagnosis labels, and insensitive attempts to do so may be disconcerting and potentially damaging to the doctor's relationship with the patient.

After the diagnosis has been presented, the doctor should be willing to explain its meaning and implications. It is likely that the patient will want a simple description of the problem, the kinds of treatment available, and an assessment of the prospect before him. However, rather than making assumptions about his wishes, it is better to invite him to ask his own questions in his own good time.

Similes and Metaphors

Although many of the problems a general practitioner must deal with are simple and straightforward, some are not and these may be difficult to explain. It may even be a problem knowing just where to begin, and here, particularly, a knowledge of the patient's own ideas gives the doctor a clear advantage.

Explanations are worthless unless they are understood, so it is important to use simple and clear language without unnecessary jargon. Patients who do not understand what is being said, or become confused, should be encouraged to interrupt and ask for clarification. Although the doctor should try not to mislead the patient, it is not necessary to be too fussy about the precise accuracy of the explanation. Scientific ideas are constantly being modified in the wake of recent advances, and in medicine it is often difficult to be dogmatic.

To explain complicated ideas analogies are helpful. Medical conditions can often be compared to everyday problems with which the patient is likely to be familiar. For example, the heart is a simple pump with one-way valves, atheromatous arteries may be likened to furred-up water pipes, and brown fat stores are radiators which burn up calories and radiate heat, and so on. Such comparisons may be inexact and not entirely satisfactory but, despite this, do not cause serious misunderstanding.

To help explain the problem it is often easier to draw a simple diagram which can be executed very quickly. The type of explanation offered will depend very much on the ingenuity of the doctor and the intelligence and existing knowledge of the patient. An example is given below which may be used to explain the symptoms of lumbago and sciatica.

Example:
Lumbago—illustrated by a drawing or a three-dimensional model.

I think the cause of your backache is disc trouble. What does this mean?

The spine is a column of bones, called vertebrae, which are separated from each other by discs. The bones are, of course, hard and relatively brittle, whereas the discs are rubbery and act as shock absorbers. Each disk is made up of a soft middle covered by several layers of gristle, rather like the layers of an onion. These give the disc its rubbery consistency. Covering the outside is a tough fibrous skin which is attached to the vertebrae and holds the whole thing in place.

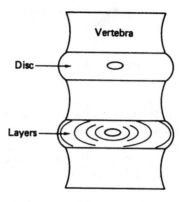

Fig. 11.1

A disc may be damaged, when the back is wrenched by lifting awkwardly or from a sudden jolt. Curiously there is often a delay between the injury and the onset of backache. Why is this, and what happens to cause the pain?

Some time after the injury, the disc or part of it loses its firm rubbery consistency and becomes soft, like creamy toothpaste, rather in the same way that an apple can change when bruised. How or why this happens remains unknown, but perhaps chemicals released from the damaged disc soften it and at the same time irritate the nerves in the disc, resulting in pain.

The spinal cord is a bundle of nerves running from the brain down the spine. It carries information like wires carry electricity.

At every vertebra a nerve emerges from the spinal cord and divides into two branches, one that goes to the disc and the other to an area of skin over the back, somewhat lower and away from the position of the disc. When the brain receives painful messages along this nerve from the disc, it thinks they have come, instead, from the area of skin, probably because skin is good at picking up sensations and this will be where such messages to the brain usually arise.

Because of this you feel your pain over a wide area of your back and not just in your spine, and that is why you may think it has originated from the muscles of your back.

This condition is called acute disc degeneration and the pain you feel is called lumbago.

What does the medical profession do for this type of backache?

This is an injury and, like most injuries, will heal on its own. The soft toothpaste-like substance of the disc eventually hardens again. Doctors can give you painkillers, which merely ease the pain, but do not heal the

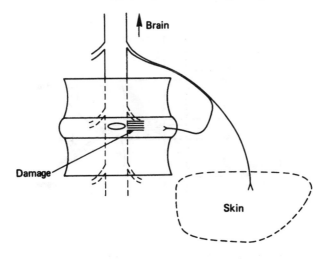

Fig. 11.2

injury. This eventually heals itself and most of the pain will disappear in about 3 weeks. In the meanwhile you should avoid further jolts to your back to prevent making it worse.

Now you know all this, do you want me to write you a prescription for any pain killers, or can you manage without or with the ones you have already?

Sciatica—(the previous explanation may be modified to suit this).

While some of the disc is still soft, there is a risk of squeezing some of the toothpaste-like substance out through a weakness in the tough fibrous skin which covers the disc. This is what has happened to you and it is called a slipped or prolapsed disc. The common problem with such an injury is that it may trap or irritate one of the nerves emerging from the spinal cord. Since this forms part of the sciatic nerve, which travels down the leg, the pain which results is called sciatica.

This nerve is not to be confused with the other nerve which was previously mentioned and that supplies the disc, although for a short distance near the spine, both nerves run alongside each other.

What should be done about a slipped disc?

If we deal with the problem early, before the damaged disc hardens up, it may be possible to ease the prolapsed disc back and free the trapped nerve.

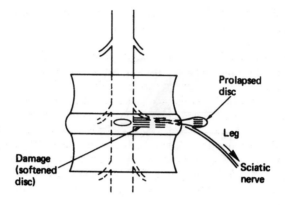

Fig. 11.3

Just as a blob of toothpaste sticking out of a toothpaste tube may be sucked back in by gently manipulating the tube of toothpaste, so with manipulation of the back. There are various ways this can be done, either by stretching it using traction, or manipulations by a physiotherapist, chiropractor or osteopath. With luck this can be very effective, resulting in rapid relief of the sciatica, although the lumbago may remain for some time after.

I hope this helps you understand what has happened, and why seemingly conflicting advice is given to people with backache, namely that some are told to rest and others are sent for manipulation.

Not all explanations need be as long as this example, indeed some may be extremely brief. However, when the problem is likely to give rise to prolonged and recurring symptoms, it is well worthwhile providing a more detailed explanation. By knowing what to expect, the patient is less likely to be alarmed with what would otherwise be unforeseen developments. He is, therefore, less likely to bother the doctor with unnecessary worries in the future. A second example is given below.

Example:
Asthma—to emphasize the importance of treating moderate asthma with an additional anti-inflammatory rather than solely a bronchodilator.

The airways of your lungs are like an upside-down hollow tree. The individual branches are tubes with an inner tube and an outer tube rather like a bicycle tyre. The outer tube of the airway is made of circular muscle, which goes into spasm during an acute attack of wheezing. Salbutamol eases this.

The inner tube is a sort of waste disposal mechanism. It produces a sticky mucous lining which traps dust, germs and pollen which you have breathed in. It also has on its surface millions of little hairy processes which waft rhythmically like the legs of a millipede, moving the mucus and trapped unwanted particles upwards and out of the lungs.

In acute asthmatic attacks this inner tube is also affected by becoming inflamed and congested. More mucus is produced, overloading the little hairs and clogging up the airways. This, together with spasm of the outer tube, prevents fresh air getting into the lungs. Even when spasm is relieved, if the inner tube is still clogged, fresh air cannot get in, nor waste air out.

Salbutamol eases only spasm. It does not act on the clogging of the inner tube. To relieve this you need to use an anti-inflammatory spray as well. This takes a few days to work, unlike Salbutamol which takes a few minutes, so it is important for you to carry on using it even though it may not at first seem to be doing any good.

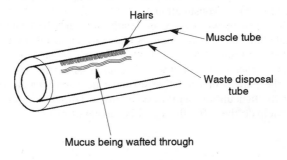

Fig. 11.4

Such explanations are not intended to be comprehensive but do provide the patient with some information to help him understand the main problems. They also enable him to ask more informed questions, which hopefully will correct any of his previous misconceptions.

Levy and others have demonstrated that from a number of items patients will remember best those pieces of information they have received first. Consequently, they advocate that doctors should give details of treatment which they regard as being more important, before offering any other advice or explanation. In situations where the doctor himself wishes to make all the decisions about treatment such advice is reasonable, but for those wishing to involve the patient in the decisions it would be inappropriate. How can patients be expected to make informed decisions without first considering the problems? Furthermore, doctors committed to involving patients do improve their patients' recollections of the consultation by encouraging them to contribute in this way.

Some doctors no doubt feel that the problem of how to treat should be decided entirely by themselves. However, others would consider this view is too exclusive, for there are many occasions where patients can safely be offered a choice of treatment and where the doctor will find himself writing fewer prescriptions as a result (Medawar, 1984). It may be surprising for some doctors to discover how few patients want prescriptions and how many would be satisfied solely with an adequate explanation of their symptoms.

Complicated problems which require involved explanations may be difficult to understand, and it may not be possible for patients to appreciate all the implications. In these circumstances the patient should not feel rushed into making ill-considered decisions, but is best asked to return at a later occasion after giving the problem some thought. He may also be invited to jot down any further questions he may wish to have answered at the next consultation.

Of course, there will be some situations where the problem is so complicated that the patient would probably never be able to understand it, or where he prefers to rely upon the doctor's judgement. There are also serious problems where it would be unfair and perhaps even upsetting for the patient or a relative to make decisions which would be emotionally difficult for them. In such circumstances the doctor should try to anticipate the difficulties and be prepared to take the responsibility.

Booklets and Explanatory Leaflets

A common impression that doctors have of patients is that they seldom like to leave the surgery empty-handed, which is possibly why general practitioners so commonly terminate their interviews by handing over prescriptions, and why consultants dispatch patients with request forms for investigations. Interestingly I have noticed how often patients ask to keep the simple drawings which have helped me to explain their problems. Among other things, they wish to use them to help pass on the information to their relatives.

Printed pamphlets which provide the patient with information are certainly very useful and have been advocated by many (Strube, 1984; Gardner, 1985). There are now a great number freely available on a wide variety of medical topics, and these make a useful addition to the doctor's own explanations. However, they are not an adequate substitute. The explanation offered by the doctor to the patient is personal and forms an essential part of reassurance, whereas printed leaflets, no matter how informative, do not. The satisfactory solution is to provide both.

Information and Investigation

Physical examination, even in general practice, is frequently supplemented by investigations. Although patients have nowadays come to accept this as usual, to many it is still a source of considerable anxiety. Since some investigations are uncomfortable and even possibly risky, it is important to involve patients in deciding whether or not to perform them. To help with their decision they should be told why the investigation is being proposed, what it would entail, and what useful information would be gained by it.

The decision to involve patients may sometimes be difficult, furthermore, misjudgement by the doctor can be upsetting, so it is important to assess the patient's feelings correctly. This is yet another reason why the doctor should be familiar with the patient's own ideas about his illness and the extent of his anxiety.

If a patient is genuinely worried that he has a possible illness which can be easily excluded by a simple investigation, then it seems sensible to carry it out, even though the doctor might consider the patient's suggestion improbable. The effect of doing so can be particularly reassuring to the patient, and a negative result will often relieve his fears instantly. Attempts at reassurance without such investigation are not usually so effective.

In contrast, patients with hypochondriasis should not be treated in this manner, although there is often a great temptation for the doctor to do so, in the hope that providing a negative result will convince the patient that his fears are unfounded; it rarely does. Instead, repeated investigations often feed the patient's growing conviction that his symptoms are organic, and this merely worsens his problem.

Prescriptions and Placebos

The ease with which patients recall information depends on how well they understand what they are told. It is, therefore, imperative that instructions about treatment should be clear and simple. Complicated information may be difficult to remember and is best written down and handed to the patient. If the doctor is unsure that the patient has understood, it is wise to repeat the instructions and then to ask the patient to recall them.

The success of any drug will depend upon its pharmacological action, the patient's belief in its effectiveness, and the degree to which he complies with the prescribed instructions. Patients are more likely to take medicines correctly if they feel that the doctor has listened and fully understood their problems. They need to feel confident in his abilities and in his diagnosis, and be convinced that his reasons for prescribing the medicine are valid. The placebo effect of any treatment is mainly due to this feeling of confidence.

The fulfilment of these criteria is one of the main functions of the consultation and it is largely this that determines the patient's satisfaction when a prescription is given.

What of the Outlook?

Many conditions are more of a temporary nuisance than a cause for serious concern, yet the patient may view the prospect quite differently and, being worried, deliberately avoid asking for reassurance. Doctors can only be fully aware of their patients' fears if they have taken the trouble to enquire about them. This emphasizes yet again the importance of this aspect of the consultation. By correcting the patients' views of their problems, the doctor will often be able to restore their peace of mind, but if he remains ignorant of them, another opportunity for reassurance will be lost.

In contrast, of course, some illnesses do not have such a favourable outlook and for a few it will be very bleak indeed. Only by discovering what the patient knows already, will the doctor be able to deal with the situation appropriately. Great care must be taken when providing patients with information which may lead them to discover further facts which they would rather not know. It is preferable to allow them to ask questions in their own good time. The doctor should try to anticipate the direction of inquiry and keep assessing the patient's intentions. Some may inadvertently ask a question which, with hindsight, they may wish they had not. These are most prudently answered by reflecting the question back to the patient until the doctor is in a better position to judge the patient's real intentions. Whatever the opinion of the doctor about such matters, his main obligation is not to harm, *primum non nocere*.

It is possible to be honest and yet avoid destroying the patient's ability to be optimistic. After all, prognostication is little more than informed guess work and, as all doctors know, exceptions to medical expectations are not rare. Apropos of this, Sir James Mackenzie made the apt, though not entirely serious remark that 'no doctor lives long enough to write a reliable book on prognosis'.

Despite considerable advances in modern therapeutics and an ever increasing amount of medical information available to the general public, there is still a widespread fear associated with malignant disease which, in many instances, is disproportionate and sometimes even grossly exaggerated. To many people cancer is equated with certain death, yet there are many types of malignancy where such a gloomy prospect is a thing of the past. If the patient is aware of the diagnosis, it is important to discover what he has already found out for himself. For many, an up-to-date prognosis will help to restore a good deal of optimism. When providing such important information as this, it is also worth including the patient's relatives, so that they will have some common ground upon which to base their future conversations together. This will prevent much unnecessary deception, which is often bewildering, and which causes so much uncertainty and suffering.

Whether to be guarded or to talk openly, whether to be truthful or to tell lies will depend very much upon the patient and the doctor's own convictions, but a great deal of help with this decision may be obtained by interviewing the patient's relatives. When the outlook becomes very poor and death seems inevitable, it is necessary to see the patient regularly and frequently. He should be allowed to direct the conversation in any direction he chooses and, as with psychotherapy, the doctor's main role is to listen. Although the patient should be given ample opportunity to ask questions, he should be left in ignorance if he so wishes, and not be nudged into avenues of inquiry he would rather avoid. However, if the doctor is sure of the patient's intentions, and the patient asks for an honest opinion about his future, it is important to be truthful, yet still endeavour to allow some room for optimism.

In contrast, where patients show strong and persistent denial, it is cruel to destroy their psychological defences by confronting them with the information they are desperately trying to evade. Without resorting to platitudes, it is quite possible to help the patient concentrate his thoughts upon the less dispiriting aspects of his illness.

Whatever decision is finally reached about this difficult problem, it is a great consolation to the patient and his relatives when the doctor makes himself easily available and is prepared to spend time with them. For situations where therapy has little chance of success, the least the doctor can do is to offer himself. By being there and by encouraging the patient to talk about his feelings, and by listening sympathetically, he can help overcome those barriers in communication that often build up between the patient and those around him. By spending time and by showing his commitment and genuine concern the general practitioner may do a great deal to improve the patient's predicament and help his relatives through their ordeal.

Chapter 12

Terminating the Consultation

'Thank you, doctor, for listening. It has helped.' Parting words by a
patient, 1984

Ideally, consultations should be concluded only when patient and doctor
are both satisfied with what has been achieved. However, not surprisingly, because they wish to keep to time, doctors often terminate their
interviews before the patient expects it. The usual way in which general
practitioners do this is by handing over a prescription. They assume,
often mistakenly, that the patient has come for a prescription and the
easiest way of removing him from the surgery is to give him one as
quickly and appropriately as possible. Unfortunately this placebo
usually pleases the patient less than the doctor hopes. Instead the patient
quite rightly has the impression that he is being pushed out. Some are
willing to accept this because their doctor is busy, but others feel understandably indignant about it.

The basis of this problem rests partly with the different expectations
of doctors and patients, as we have seen, and partly with their own individual awareness of how quickly time is passing. To the patient a consultation will usually seem a lot shorter than to the doctor for whom it is
routine. Using a prescription as a means of terminating the consultation
is a great temptation, yet it is a poor method, often resulting in over
prescribing to dissatisfied patients. However, it is unrealistic to expect
all consultations to end well, but with a little understanding and patience
doctors could improve the present level of patient satisfaction.

Another problem which frequently occurs at the end of a consultation
is the introduction by the patient of a completely new set of symptoms.
This 'by the way ...' phenomenon causes a great deal of exasperation to
all doctors, much of which is unnecessary. To avoid it, patients should
be encouraged at an early stage in the consultation to introduce all the
problems they wish to discuss. Furthermore, when they are allowed to
participate more actively they are less likely to withhold important
information. If, however, an additional problem does arise unexpectedly
in this way, it is obvious that the patient must have been reluctant to
talk about it previously. So it is important not to discourage him as it
is likely to be of major concern. If put off, particularly in a manner that
the patient might consider brusque, the opportunity to talk about it may
be lost permanently.

When there is not enough time available to deal effectively with the problem, the patient should be told that what he wants to say is obviously important and needs to be discussed in further detail. An early appointment should be offered and a note made in the records reminding the doctor about it next time.

Usually there is little difficulty in terminating consultations, but occasionally patients are so preoccupied and self-absorbed that they are insensitive to the usual cues telling them that their interview is over. They have to be told firmly and politely, and sometimes even taken by the arm and escorted to the door. Such patients may be amusing to talk about to colleagues but are rarely so amusing to have in the surgery. However, it is seldom worth becoming annoyed with them as their insensitivity prevents them from appreciating the doctor's point of view.

Perhaps surprisingly, some doctors have difficulty in terminating their consultations and regularly overrun their appointment times. They fail to draw the interview to a succinct conclusion and the patient remains unaware of any sense of achievement from the consultation. Failing in this, they frequently distract themselves and their patients with further random questions upon topics which should have been previously covered, but which were unfortunately omitted. This usually leaves the patient thoroughly confused.

A good history draws to a conclusion naturally. It must be easily anticipated by the patient, who then feels satisfied to leave with a clear idea of the subsequent course of action that he will have to take.

Formalizing the process of conclusion is one of the unexpected benefits of computerization, and for this reason I have delayed mention of it until now.

Before the introduction of computers into my own practice, I used to refrain from taking notes until the patient had left the room, as I felt my time was better served by observing and listening throughout. I still feel this is the preferred option, but if computers are to be used for clinical records, and I realize the many advantages of this, the choice of medication should be linked with it. In which case, there is no alternative but to type in at least the heading entry first, and then issue the prescription. This obviously has to be done in the patient's presence.

I do not intend to describe how to use a computer, as this has been done in detail elsewhere (Preece 1994; Sheldon and Stodart 1985) and in any event would be well beyond the brief of this book. However, I would like to mention how it may be used beneficially and with the minimum of intrusion.

Computer Records

The last decade has brought many changes into general practice: fundholding, videorecording and computerization are but three. Despite my own initial reservations about the intrusion that computers would have upon the consultation and my fears that it would result in some measure of depersonalization, I have grown to realize their great merits. As with any implement, the manner in which it is used, rather than the device itself, determines its success or failure. Computers themselves are not alienating, only the way in which they are deployed, often by the intellectually insecure in their impoverished attempt to exclude the uninitiated.

The great benefit that computers provide is the storage and retrieval of information, but this is of value only if the information entered is accurate and stored in an orderly manner. For those unfamiliar with using a computer, and for those who use one badly, it is important to realize that its potential depends ultimately upon the user. Put rubbish in and all you will get out is rubbish, albeit neatly stored, but completely useless.

It is vital from the outset that the user has a clear, simple idea of how to enter information, so that it is easily accessible and intelligible, not only for himself but for any other rightful user. It is possible to enter any amount of detail but unless it is stored in the right places it will be very time consuming to find at a later date.

Furthermore, searches for data for the purposes of audit will be difficult if not impossible if the information is not properly entered. Time spent at this early stage will save so much wasted effort later on.

Since time in general practice is always pressing, and audit and computerization are becoming increasingly important, the ability to use a keyboard is a growing requirement. This not only speeds up the time taken for the doctor to make his notes, but also reduces the interference that this has upon the consultation. It is certainly worth learning how to type.

Whatever your technique, whether it be that of a 60 word per minute touch typist or a pedestrian 'hunt and peck' lurcher, your records should still be orderly and accurate. Care to ensure this is time well spent.

Before you can type anything into the clinical records, you must first select a coded reference. Often you will choose the patient's presenting symptom, e.g. breathlessness, or you may choose a diagnostic category, e.g. LVF, provided that you are already sure of this. Once you have selected this heading which will already be in the computer's memory under a Read Code Number, you are then presented with two main options:

either 1 *Prescription:* You may decide to type nothing further in front of the patient, but instead immediately issue a prescription. Once this has been printed and handed to the patient, you may bid him farewell and then continue making further notes. However, you may type 'free text' (whatever you wish) only when you have entered in another coded heading, on which to add your 'free text'.

or 2 *Clinical Notes:* You may prefer, however, to complete your clinical notes before finally deciding on your course of action, e.g. a prescription or referral or advice. To do this, however, means that the patient will remain whilst you do so. Should the VDU be hidden from his view and you take time to key in your entries, the patient may become exasperated, annoyed or worried. With increased emphasis upon patient autonomy and cooperation, it is preferable in most instances to allow him to see what you are typing and involve him albeit passively in this part of the consultation. By asking the patient if what you have written accords with his own thoughts, you will reduce the risk of dispute or disagreement later on, should the patient demand to see his records.

For those who have not yet involved patients in this way, and therefore remain apprehensive of it, I would like to reassure them that there is little to feel threatened about, and indeed the whole experience is usually mutually beneficial.

The advantages of the first option is the speed with which the consultation is terminated, and the minimal intrusion into the consultation that the computer makes. Furthermore, information which might be worrying for the patient is withheld until he has left the room.

The advantages of the second option is the greater involvement of the patient in the doctor's record keeping. He can see exactly what is written and he does not feel excluded. He sees conclusions reinforced in print, and he can observe that diagnoses applied to him are recognized categories, stored within the computer's memory and not something nebulous shrouded in unintelligible jargon that the doctor has just made up. He feels much closer to being a 'Partner in Care'.

Whichever option is chosen the strict logical process of the computer instils into the procedure a disciplined formality which clearly punctuates the final phase of the consultation.

On pressing the final key the printer spurts into action to complete the process. The doctor rises to tear off the prescription, presenting the patient with an indelible cue to rise also and accept it from the doctor, who opens the door for the patient to depart.

The expectation of the patient is upset only if he has further problems he wishes to have aired. For this reason it is so important for the doctor to have tackled all the patient's problems beforehand, so avoiding that final common offering, 'Oh, by the way ...'.

Chapter 13

Video Assessment

> 'Over the past few years we have introduced many general practice
> trainees and principals—both trainers and doctors not involved in
> training—to the delights of seeing themselves on video. Nearly all of
> these doctors were very apprehensive about the experience before-
> hand. It must be remembered that, while there is anxiety about the
> recording of consultations, apprehension is probably greater about
> showing the recording to a group of peers'.
>
> Pendleton, Schofield, Tate and Havelock
> *The Consultation—An Approach to Learning and Teaching, 1984*

Over the last ten years the video market has expanded and become
commonplace. Video recorders are present in most schools, and the
videotape has become one of the most powerful and useful teaching
aids to be introduced this century. With easy availability of small and
affordable video cameras of good quality, most GP Registrars have
been encouraged to record themselves during their consultations, to
view them critically with their trainers, and so modify and improve
their technique.

One of the great benefits that recording has brought, is to enable
the same consultation to be viewed time and time again. Gestures and
incidents, which could easily be overlooked on first inspection, can
be pinpointed, providing a unique opportunity for appraisal and
development.

In the first edition of my book in 1986 then entitled *Partners in Care*,
I offered the suggestion that the Royal College of General Practitioners
(RCGP) might include in its Membership Examination an assessment of
the candidate's consultation technique. Several others in the profession
held the same view, and so convincing were the arguments that such
scrutiny is now to be included both in this examination and in
Summative Assessment for all young GPs wishing to become principals.

No doubt as a potential candidate you will be nervous about the
prospect of recording yourself on tape, so one of the purposes of this new
edition is to reassure and encourage you, and to help prepare yourself for
this. How then should you begin?

Preparation

First, before you start to record yourself, look at as many video consultations of others as you can. There are a few available and no doubt your Course Organizer and your Trainer will help you in your search. In 1986 the Royal Society of Medicine produced an excellent series of ten videotapes. These were produced in association with the Department of General Practice at the University of Liverpool and were entitled *Problems in Doctor/Patient Encounters—Learning from one another*. Although these are rather expensive to buy they can be obtained through your local Postgraduate Medical Centre Library. In addition, the MSD Foundation, then headed by Marshall Marinker, also produced a series of video consultations, called 'Brief Encounters', by different doctors of varying experience demonstrating different styles and techniques. These were released on one tape. Unfortunately, however, the MSD Foundation has ceased to exist but copies of the tape are still available, and may be obtained through your library.

Many Course Organizers encourage their GP Registrars to bring video consultations of themselves to the VTS workshops, and no doubt, because of the new regulations this will be encouraged even more.

In this way you should be able to familiarize yourself with some of the many ways in which GPs conduct their consultations. You may recognize some similarities in the way that you yourself consult. You may gain insight about techniques that so far you have avoided. Some things you will criticize and disapprove of, and feel that you could do better. Either way there will be many opportunities for you to broaden your experiences and learn from your colleagues.

Role play may be used to good effect, especially when actors are employed as patients (Field, Jeffrey and Wright, 1995), and provides yet another lively way to improve consultation skills. Every chance should be seized beforehand to anticipate the problems ahead. Remember, it is good practice, whenever you consult, to imagine observing yourself whilst doing so. This use of the 'video in the head' is a practice that will be valuable to you for all your professional life. In your training year, before the pressure of being a principal begins, you should make the most of your opportunities. At first it may take time to collect your thoughts between consultations, to reflect about what you have done and how you have achieved it. Keeping a diary is a good habit to adopt. Stott, in 1983, in his book *Milestones, the Diary of a Trainee GP*, kept an excellent record of the whole of his Trainee year. He focused particularly on the psychological aspects of general practice. You could do likewise and also direct your attention at the ways misunderstandings arise and how better understanding is achieved. You could observe and record the occasions when fleeting mood changes pass over the patient's face, and consider the sort of questions that brought them about. You could reflect upon the occasions when vital cues were missed, and how, had you behaved differently, the outcome would have changed.

All the time you will be improving both your clinical skill and your powers of observation. You will also be aware of your own feelings. Record them as well and try to identify the reasons for their arousal. Were they to do with your reaction to the patient, or were they a throw back to another situation and someone else of whom the patient reminded you? This is particularly useful if your feelings are strong.

Everything should be recorded in your mind whilst you consult. This concept of the 'video in the head', that I described in the first edition, has been since extensively developed by Neighbour as the 'Inner Consultation'.

Initially you may be disturbed to find your clinical thoughts distracted by your reflections about the consultation process. Do not be discouraged, with practice it will become easier.

When recording yourself on video, I would recommend that you keep your technique simple, listen well, and restrict your enquiry to a few, clear, considered questions. Try to make your history-taking all of a piece, before you move to the examination and subsequent offers of explanation and treatment. It is just as confusing for you, the patient and your assessors if you dart back and forth, eliciting different aspects of the story at random.

Try also to trust your memory, and your mind's ability to do the sorting of information, while the patient speaks. Have the confidence to look at the patient and listen rather than record his answers immediately they are uttered. Patients often modify their answers after further consideration, and so much valuable information may be lost in those brief periods of distraction, if you are for ever writing in the notes.

For the majority who make handwritten notes, record taking can be done without diversion and with far better concentration, once the patient has left the room. For those growing number who use computerized records, however, this is not possible without 'unlinking' the clinical entry from the prescribed medication. This is one of the undoubted disadvantages of the computer, which otherwise provides many benefits. To link the clinical record with the prescribed medication it is necessary first to key in the clinical data before issuing the prescription and so must be done in the patient's presence.

Nevertheless whether or not you use a computer, try to wait until the end of the consultation before making your notes. In this way, as you turn your attention away from the patient, and excuse yourself whilst you do so, you may draw the consultation to its natural conclusion. For those doctors who have difficulty in terminating their consultations this is a useful technique. To this end also, the computer printer does offer an additional air of finality which helps conclude the interview.

As you will have already seen, this has been discussed in greater detail in the previous chapter: Terminating the Consultation.

The main aim in producing a video of the consultation is to try as best as one can to conduct an honest exploration of the patient's presenting complaints, avoiding distortion and harmful error. In providing a video-recording therefore, the GP Registrar would do well to remember a few simple points:

1   Have faith in your own consulting style. Undoubtedly through the course of your professional life you will mature, and with that maturity your technique of questioning and listening will change. This metamorphosis will be a blend of your own character, your clinical skill, and your own experience of life. Later on particularly, it also includes other less desirable factors such as declining memory, inattentiveness and impatience.

In the meantime you have so far spent several years developing your technique. It will not be perfect, because no technique ever is. But do look at it critically to ensure that it is neither inappropriate nor potentially harmful.

2   Don't expect to produce the best video recording on your first attempt. Try a few preliminary runs, and look at the better tapes with your trainer before choosing the best one to send off for assessment.

3   Give the patient and yourself adequate time for each consultation. If all you do on the tape is issue hurried sick notes, and prescribe antibiotics for sore throats, it is unlikely to impress the assessors. You will not be giving them sufficient evidence of your competence, so do not sell yourself short.

4   Make sure that the quality of the recording is adequate. The lighting should be directed at the faces of both doctor and patient. Avoid placing the camera facing a window, as the doctor and patient will then be seen only in silhouette. Most importantly the sound should be of good quality, so that everything that is said by both parties can be easily heard. Clearly this will not be possible when you move away from the camera to an examination room, but the assessors know full well that it is unfair and unrealistic to expect patients to allow you to record the examination.

5   Your understanding of the strengths and weaknesses of each consultation will be something that the assessors will be marking. It is, therefore, important to view your video critically and record your ideas and reservations clearly in your accompanying log.

Recording Details

When submitting video material for Summative Assessment, you will be required to provide approximately twelve consultations on two hours of continuous VHS tape (standard play). A visual timer display will have to be provided on the tape, or alternatively a clock may be placed in view of the camera throughout the recording.

Remember it is unrealistic to expect that you will achieve both a satisfactory surgery of consultations and a good quality recording with your first attempt. Be prepared for several, and do expect to be disappointed, alarmed, even amused or possibly all three. Anyone who has videoed himself, will have experienced a variety of such feelings when watching himself for the first time, so you should not be disheartened. The experience will undoubtedly make you a better doctor.

Equipment

For recording you will need a well-lit room, a videocamera for VHS tape, a tripod, a clock or intrinsic timer on the videocamera, sufficient tape for two hours' recording, and ideally an external extension microphone complete with stand. Whilst it is possible to use small cassette tapes which fit into the camera, these last only about three-quarters of an hour and you would therefore have two interruptions to change tapes in order to provide two hours of continuous recording. To obviate this you can connect most cameras directly to a standard videorecorder and record on a three-hour tape, which is so much easier.

Videocamera

This should be easily portable complete with tripod, unless the surgery to which you are attached has built-in videomonitor equipment. It should be of the VHS mode with a wide angle lens. Most doctors' consulting rooms are small and such a lens is necessary in order to get both patient and doctor into view and in reasonable close-up. Most modern cameras have such a built-in facility. Even despite this, it may not be possible to fit both the face of the patient and that of the doctor into the frame. In this case, an oblique view with the camera slightly behind the doctor's shoulder and directed at the patient's face is the best compromise.

Most cameras have both a 'standard play' and 'long play' option. Some cameras will take a normal three-hour tape, but most use compact cassettes which last 45 minutes. By altering the setting to 'long play' these small cassettes will extend their playing time to about one and a half hours. To view them, however, you will need a recorder with a similar facility, and the tape you finally submit will have to be recorded on standard play. To achieve this, you will have to have a videorecorder capable of performing this transformation.

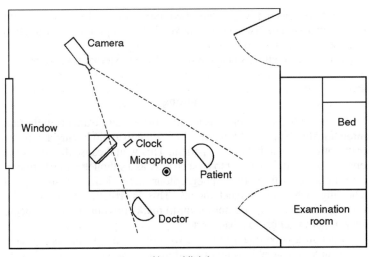

Natural lighting

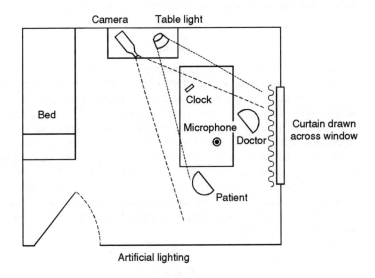

Artificial lighting

Fig. 13.1

It is possible to link most cameras to a videorecorder as I mentioned previously and this is probably the simplest way of obtaining two hours of recording. This not only avoids the interruptions of tape changes, but also the irritation of discovering that you have lost part of a consultation because the tape has run out.

The camera should also have a socket for an external microphone.

Lighting

Try to ensure that the lighting is good. Most modern cameras will adapt automatically to poor light, but it is important to avoid having a window or bright table lamp behind the patient. This would cause the iris of the lens to close, and the subject to be seen only as a silhouette. Furthermore, poor lighting will produce poor colour definition, and subsequent 'ghosting' when the subject moves. This is irritating to watch, and although the assessors are not meant to mark film quality, it is prudent for you not to get off to a bad start.

To obtain a good quality picture with the minimum of fuss, place a light source (e.g. a table lamp or window) behind the camera so that the light is directed at the patient's face. If there is no alternative to seating the patient in front of a window, draw the curtains and illuminate the patient with appropriate artificial lighting (see Fig. 13.1).

Sound

Most cameras have a built-in microphone, and if the camera is placed close to the patient and both doctor and patient speak clearly, the sound recording can be quite good. So often, however, patients speak softly, whilst doctors, perhaps in order to compensate, frequently shout. This causes distortion and is irritating to listen to. To avoid missing important details within the consultation, you may use an extension microphone of good quality, placed in a stand on the desk equidistant from patient and doctor. A stand is important because without one, it is so easy to pick up distracting noises such as the rustling of papers or tapping of pens on the desk, yet another source of irritation for the assessors. For the same reason it is best placed slightly away from any keyboard you may use.

Consent

Over the last decade there has been much ethical discussion about the use of videorecording and the consequent possible breaches of confidentiality. There has also been discussion about this in Parliament. The ethics and acceptability of videorecording have been well described in Chapter 9 of Pendleton's now classic text *The Consultation: An*

PATIENT'S CONSENT FORM AND INFORMATION SHEET—SUMMATIVE ASSESSMENT

Patient's name ....

Consent to Video Recording for Assessment Purposes

❏ We are hoping to make video recordings of some of the consultations between patients and

  Doctor .... whom you are seeing today.

❏ The videos are for part of an assessment procedure designed to make sure that all doctors who become GPs are fully competent.

❏ The video is ONLY of you and the doctor talking together. No intimate examination will be done in front of the camera. All video recordings are carried out according to guidelines agreed by the Joint Committee on Postgraduate Training for General Practice, which is the body responsible for the training of GPs.

❏ The video will be seen only by doctors involved in assessment and training of general practice trainees, the tape will then be erased. The tape will be stored in a locked cabinet and is subject to the same degree of confidentiality and security as medical records. The Regional Assessment Committee will be responsible for storage of the tape. The tape will be erased as soon as practicable and in any event within 1 year. The results of this work may be used for research and educational purposes.

❏ You do not have to agree to your consultation with the doctor being recorded. If you want the camera turned off, please tell Reception—this is not a problem, and will not affect your consultation in any way.

❏ But if you do not mind your consultation being recorded, we are grateful to you. Improving the assessment of GPs should lead to a better service to patients.

❏ If you wish you may view the tape recording.

❏ If you consent to this consultation being recorded, please sign below. Thank you very much for your help.

Signed.. Date ....

Signature(s) of any accompanying person (s) ....

❏ After you have finished seeing the doctor, please sign below to confirm that you are still happy to have the recording used.

Signed.. Date ....

For doctor's use only   Reference number:

Fig. 13.2

Approach to Learning and Teaching. The co-authors of this text have recommended the following practical points:

1 All patients must give written and informed consent on each and every occasion of recording.
2 Patients must be given every possible opportunity to refuse.
3 Written consent must include permission to record, and permission to show the video to other doctors.
4 The patient should always be given the opportunity to have the recording erased at the end of the consultation if he so wishes.

Nationally accepted consent forms for video assessment are now available and must be used on each occasion, and kept safely. Remember 'written consent from a well-informed patient is the best defence against criticism, both legal and moral'—Pendleton *et al. The Consultation.*

For your Summative Assessment, combined patient consent forms and information sheets will be provided. An example may be seen in Fig. 13.2.

Tips for Taping

Before you begin your recording it is worth considering a few important practical points:

1 *Appointments:* You are expected to produce 12 video consultations on the two-hour tape. Appointments, therefore, should be booked every ten minutes. It is important, within a reasonable degree of flexibility to try and keep to this schedule.
2 *Clock:* Remember to face the clock to the camera, to ensure it is working properly and that it tells the correct time.
3 *Housekeeping:* Neighbour uses this term referring to those feelings in ourselves, such as exasperation, anger or sadness, that may linger on from previous consultations or events. It is important for your wellbeing and that of the patient that they don't spill over into the next consultation, and adversely affect the outcome. 'House-keeping' may also embrace other more mundane considerations which, if neglected, could also cause problems. For example, before the next patient walks into the room, you should have finished recording your previous findings, either in the handwritten notes, or on the computer. All the paper records should be placed neatly back into the folder, and if the patient is to be referred, those notes should be appropriately tagged or placed in the correct basket awaiting referral. If a computer is used, the previous patient's records must be removed from the screen before the next patient enters. A video record of serious errors possibly involving breaches

of confidence will not create a favourable impression with the assessors. In fact it will probably result in your failure.

At the beginning of the next consultation, as the patient enters, be ready to greet him by name, and match him with the correct records. At the same time thank him for agreeing to be videoed, and briefly give him the opportunity to withdraw his consent.

4 *Manner:* Remember, try to make your manner unaffected. You want the patient and yourself to behave as naturally as possible. Neither of you should be camera shy nor playing to the gallery. An honest record is required, not a melodrama.

If you have noticed in previous recordings that you have developed a distracting habit, such as fiddling with a pen, try to eradicate it. Perhaps you could gently grasp the arm of your chair with your dominant hand?

5 *Listen:* Do allow the patient sufficient time to voice his presenting complaints. Listen carefully to what is said and the way it is said, and refrain from rushing in with premature questions. Much may be surmised from the patient's choice of opening gambit (Neighbour, 1987), his use of words and his gestures. Whilst some of this may be lost in the videorecording, you may make useful reference to it in your accompanying log, when appropriate to do so, to create a favourable impression.

Try to confine yourself to a few well-directed enquiries and be sure to listen to the answers. It will not look well if your next question has already just been answered.

Encourage the patient to present all his problems before you examine him. If you don't have time to deal with them all, say so courteously, and treat the most pressing problems, whilst inviting the patient to make a return appointment.

If the patient suddenly begins to unburden himself of some stressful emotional problem, you would do well to consider extending the consultation, even if this spoils your schedule. This is especially important if you feel that the patient has been suppressing his feelings for a considerable time, and, if not grasped now, the opportunity might be lost for good. Remember your prime reason for seeing the patient is to treat him well, not to produce a good recording for your assessment. A diversion from your appointment schedule in such unusual circumstances will be understandable to the assessors, and you will be able to justify it in your log.

In many situations, however, when the patient wishes to discuss difficult emotional problems, it is often easier and more suitable to offer a longer appointment at a more convenient time. This can be done tactfully and encouragingly, without affront to the patient. For example you could say: 'You've obviously got a lot of worries that you need to discuss, which might have an important bearing on your problem. I could offer you a longer appointment next week, where you would feel less rushed. How would that suit you?'

6 *Patient's Agenda:* Do not forget to ask the patient for his own thoughts, worries and conclusions about his problem. Often patients are surprised by this sort of questioning, and are initially baffled by it. You may have to provide encouragement as patients can feel a little foolish explaining their ideas to someone more knowledgeable. However, it is often most revealing, and it will help focus your remarks when you come to inform and reassure him.

7 *Examination:* When you examine the patient you will probably be out of view of the camera, and possibly out of earshot. In case important information is lost, when you are back within view of the camera, it is quite a good idea for the benefit of the assessors, to briefly sketch out your findings to the patient. Whatever you say, make it simple and accurate, taking care to avoid unnecessary distress.

8 *Explanation:* Try to begin your explanation of the problem with reference to the patient's own ideas. Correct any medical misunderstandings he may have. Recapitulate the problem to the patient to ensure you have understood it correctly. Then continue with your own explanation, restricting the use of medical words to those which you consider useful for the patient to know. The use of terminology does offer the dignity of a diagnosis and with it the hope of a recognized treatment. It may also help erase a common misapprehension felt by many patients of not being taken seriously or considered hypochondriacal.

9 *Treatment:* If you feel it applicable, involve the patient in his own management. Try to ascertain how the patient feels about the various choices open to him. In this you must be guided by your own conclusions about the patient's intellect, ability and willingness to be a 'partner in care'. Invite him to make his own choice, or alternatively ask the patient if he is content with the decision you would make for him. If the decision seems particularly difficult don't rush him. Instead, invite him back, when he has had time to consider. Offer him a leaflet on the matter and suggest he discuss it with his spouse or other relatives. Perhaps he could bring his relative along next time?

All this will be appreciated not only by the patient but by your assessors. It will demonstrate that you understand the difficulties that patients sometimes face.

10 *Conclusion of the Consultation:* After your management plan, the patient should feel the consultation drawing naturally to a close. If

you use a computer for the records, now is the time to type in your entry. The patient may be able to see what you have written, and it is perfectly reasonable to involve him in this activity. Of course, you may not yet wish to involve the patient in worrying information, in which case this may be entered separately after he has left the surgery. Remember whatever you do, you must feel able to justify it in your written log.

Issue your prescription, and if this is done through your computer, you will probably have to stand up to tear the prescription from the printer. By remaining standing whilst handing the prescription to the patient, the consultation is clearly and simply brought to a close. Furthermore it is often a good idea to open the door for the patient and either renew the invitation for a further appointment or to bid him goodbye.

11 *Housekeeping:* Once the patient has left the room, close the door, return to the computer or your notes, to make any additional entries that you feel are necessary. Then place the notes in the correct basket, or tag them suitably, using whichever system is employed to return the notes to file, or to leave them out for referral. If you use a computer, clear the record from the screen, and only then call the next patient in. However, just before you do, check how you feel and try to erase any emotional 'spillage' from the previous consultation.

The Log Book

The purpose of the log book is to provide the assessors with information which is not accessible from your videorecording, for example background information about the patient's social circumstances, or his past medical history where either of these is relevant, or the disclosure of your own thoughts and conclusions about what happened during the consultation.

These bits of information should be brief and to the point. The log entry for each consultation, therefore, should contain:

1 The candidate's name.
2 The number of the consultation.
3 The camera clock: time of commencement and duration of the consultation.
4 The reason for the patient's attendance. This might not be the immediately presenting complaint.
5 The physical findings, both positive and relevant negative ones.
6 The action taken, e.g. the prescribed treatment, information leaflet, details of referral.

7   The outline: in about 50 words you should outline the setting of the consultation, what you achieved and what issues might arise in the future.

8   Finally you should rate the degree of difficulty of the consultation as either straightforward/moderate/difficult.

To give you a better idea of how the log may relate to a consultation, the following example is provided.

Videorecording

This shows a 65-year-old man complaining of cold feet. It is apparent that he is a regular attender at the surgery, and that this is a follow-up appointment for the control of his angina, which now seems stable. Your enquiry suggests that he is not in heart failure, and he has been on Atenolol for almost a year.

Investigating the patient's own ideas reveals that he is worried about his cold feet, as this could indicate poor circulation, something he has been told could be due to his smoking.

Your examination is off screen, but on your return you reassure him that his circulation is adequate and the pulses in his feet are easily felt. You agree that his smoking could damage his circulation. Furthermore you tell him that his cold feet may be at least partly due to Atenolol, which you feel ought to be stopped and replaced by another drug, which might improve blood flow. You prescribe Isosorbide Mononitrate.

You conclude the consultation by agreeing that he ought to stop smoking and by offering him another appointment to help him deal with this.

You hand him an anti-smoking leaflet and ask him to read it for next time and hand him the prescription, giving him clear instructions how to take it.

Log book entry

Your log might read:

1   Your name
2   Third consultation out of 12
3   Time of commencement 9.22 a.m.
    Lasted 9 minutes
4   Reasons for patient's attendance:
    a   Follow-up of angina treatment (Doctor initiated)
    b   Worry about circulation to legs (Patient initiated)

5 Physical findings:
   a Normal dorsalis pedis pulses
   b No signs of heart failure
   c Sinus bradycardia 56 pm
     BP 145/85
6 Action taken:
   a Replaced Atenolol with Isosorbide Mononitrate
   b Gave leaflet about stopping smoking
7 Outline:
   A 65-year-old smoker with IHD on Atenolol. Peripheral pulses were present. Bradycardia and cold feet probably due to Atenolol. Patient's concern about smoking was addressed. He was treated appropriately and offered help with smoking. Future worries include MI, stroke and claudication. Follow-up was arranged
8 Degree of difficulty—moderate.

The MRCGP Video Assessment

The rules governing videotaped consultations and the methods by which they are assessed are somewhat different for the MRCGP examination compared with Summative Assessment. The candidate is expected to provide a videotape of between 20 to 24 consultations prepared in much the same way as for Summative Assessment. The candidate's performance, however, will be judged according to 11 criteria:

1 *Encouraging the patient's contribution:* The doctor encourages the patient to contribute by exploring his ideas and conclusions, and by involving him where appropriate in decisions about management and choices in treatment.

2 *Being alert to cues:* Patients by intention or otherwise often provide hints about problems that they might not present overtly. The doctor should not be insensitive to these important clues.

3 *Placing the complaint in its correct social and psychological context:* The doctor elicits details from the patient which enables him to place the complaint within its appropriate setting. For example a patient might present with a headache and on further questioning reveal that her husband has left home for another woman and is refusing to pay maintenance.

4 *Not missing serious conditions:* The doctor is expected to take an adequate clinical history to prevent missing serious conditions and causing grave error.

5 *Examining appropriately:* The doctor is expected to examine whatever system seems appropriate to address the patient's problem.

6   *Making the appropriate diagnosis:* The doctor's diagnosis should accord with the history and examination.

7   *Explaining the diagnosis, management and treatment:* The doctor provides an adequate explanation of the diagnosis so that the patient understands it, and can thereby give informed consent about treatment, and be involved as a partner in his own management where this is appropriate.

8   *Using language appropriate to the patient's needs:* Before the patient can give informed consent he must first understand what the doctor is saying. This should be tailored to the patient. Clearly an explanation to a patient who is a doctor would be quite different from that presented to a patient with no prior medical knowledge.

9   *Sharing management choices:* There are many instances where patients can be involved in choosing between various options in management and treatment.

10 *Appropriate prescribing:* The doctor should be expected to prescribe medication suitable for the patient's condition and diagnosis.

11 *The management plan should reflect good practice:* The doctor constructs a plan for management which demonstrates good medical practice and accords with generally accepted standards.

Clearly not all these criteria will be met in every consultation, nor would it be desirable that they should be, as this would demonstrate obsessive, inflexible behaviour. However, it is generally expected that each performance criterion should be achieved at least three times over the duration of 20 to 24 consultations.

The Workbook

As with the summative assessment, so too in the MRCGP examination, candidates will have to submit an accompanying log or workbook. This is made up of five sections:

Section 1   This is an index to the tape, giving the date and time of each consultation and a grade from 1 to 3 according to the level of difficulty, 1 being the easiest and 3 the most demanding.

Section 2   Six consultations are chosen from the total of 20 to 24 submitted. These are selected by the candidate according to whether he considers they best demonstrate the criteria that the assessors are looking for. Corresponding to a list of the eleven performance criteria will be six columns for the best consultations. In these columns the candidate indicates which criteria he thinks have been achieved.

Section 3 This part of the workbook includes forms which provide a brief assessment of all the consultations submitted. Each form will include the patient's age, sex, length and booked time of the consultation, the presenting complaint and relevant background together with the outcome. The candidate is also expected to comment on the consultation saying what he thought went well and what he might have done better.

Section 4 This section requires the candidate to provide a detailed analysis of five consultations, which is to be done in two separate ways:

a   *A minute by minute account.* The doctor must state clearly what is happening through each minute of the consultation. For example:

0–1 minute	The patient is correctly identified and welcomed. The matching notes or computer records are produced. The patient offers his opening gambit.
1–2 minutes	The patient explains that he has had a headache on and off for three days, that there is a past history of recurring headaches.
3–4 minutes	The patient acknowledges a family history of migraine.
6–7 minutes	The doctor offers an explanation of migraine and possible trigger factors.
8–9 minutes	The patient is involved in a strategy for managing his own migraine and for trying to avoid further trigger factors.

b   *'Consultation Map' charted against time.* This will show the time at which each performance criterion was achieved.

Section 5 Relevant personal details of the candidate and the practice where the consultation took place.

The Assessment

Provided that all 11 criteria are performed three times to a satisfactory standard, the videotape will be passed on its first assessment by one single examiner. If there is any doubt, the tape will be viewed by two other assessors together. Here the candidate will pass or fail. Therefore, a candidate will fail on this part of the test only after his tape has been viewed by three examiners.

This is a pass or fail test, and no success or exhibition of excellence in other parts of the examination can offset a failure in this test of consultation skill. If, however, a candidate fails here but passes in all other sections, he may submit a second tape without a further fee. Satisfaction here will result in a pass. Failure will necessitate a complete reentry, and another fee.

Final Advice

When you have finished recording your consultations and have selected the series that you feel is most satisfactory, do ask your Trainer to view it with you. It will be his eventual responsibility to ensure you are not submitting a tape that is below standard, or reveals a serious error that could harm the patient, or a succession of minor mishaps.

Remember your Trainer will not want you to fail unnecessarily as it will reflect upon him as well as on you, nor will he want to embarrass himself by allowing you to send off a tape which other assessors subsequently find unacceptable.

Chapter 14

Conclusions

'Yet the technical, academic, and administrative demands on GPs seem to grow with every report that is published about their activities and some, like some of their hospital colleagues, no longer have time to fulfil what is occasionally dismissed as their "pastoral role".

'Could it be that we need a special doctor just to guide patients through our complex medical world, to protect their interests, sustain their spirit and, like the hospice doctors, use science and skill to care for all of us who are dying, though the imminence of our deaths is less predictable than it is for the hospice patient.

'We used to have such doctors. They were called GPs. Today's bearers of that title are subjected to a form of "vocational training" much praised by those who organize it. Indeed, postgraduate training for doctors is now more complex and more organized than it has ever been, yet increasing numbers of intelligent, rational people ... have to search outside orthodox medicine, often fishing in waters that they don't find particularly savoury, in their desperate attempts to find someone to sustain the spirit in the way that doctors once used to do.'
Michael O'Donnell—*Doctor! Doctor! An Insider's Guide to the Games Doctors Play*

In the 1950s general practice was the Cinderella service of the newly formed tripartite National Health Service. GPs found themselves inundated by patients wanting the new 'free' service and not surprisingly surgeries were hopelessly overcrowded. Patients often had to sit for hours in packed waiting rooms, not knowing how long it would be before their turn to see the doctor would come. Because the flood gates had been well and truly opened, nothing but the briefest of consultations could be offered. Yet the increased demand and the amount of hidden illness that it revealed placed an enormous strain upon those doctors who felt committed to making it work. As an additional source of exasperation, free access to the hospital service meant that GPs were expected to refer many patients they would otherwise have treated themselves, had they sufficient time.

Secretaries and receptionists were by no means as common as they are today and, in consequence, notes were poorly kept and sometimes badly filed, appointments non-existent, and referral letters often skimped probably because they were handwritten.

By the early 1960s the system was nearing collapse and many dissatisfied doctors found it easier to emigrate than stay to face a future that seemed increasingly unattractive.

The rift between specialists and general practitioners grew wider and as technology began to be introduced into modern medicine it grew wider still. Teaching hospital consultants seemed to have a generally poor opinion of GPs and made no effort to conceal their feelings when talking to medical students. Morale certainly was extremely low, and it even seemed possible that general practice might disappear altogether to be replaced by an all-specialist system.

Fortunately however, 'The Doctors' Charter', worked out between 1964 and 1966, brought about substantial reforms which have continued over the last 20 years. Improved organization, open access to laboratory and hospital facilities, fairer division of work and pay, and improved status have all contributed to make general practice an attractive future for newly qualified doctors. This has increased the competition for GP posts and, together with compulsory training, has improved the standard of newly appointed principals.

General practice has been revived, yet numerous surveys and reports still suggest that more improvements are needed. Patients often complain that their doctors fail to listen or to understand what they are trying to say, and doctors frequently become irritated with patients who bother them with trivialities. This mutual dissatisfaction must be a result of inadequate communication, and over the last 10 years researchers have tried to analyse what the GP does or attempts to do during his consultations.

More recently, audio and video tape recordings of real consultations have enabled an even closer scrutiny, and these, together with role-play, are frequently used to teach new doctors the techniques of interviewing. Nevertheless, there are still very few books published, written by general practitioners, which attempt to teach those aspects of the consultation that set the general practitioner apart from his specialist medical colleagues. I hope then, that this book makes some contribution.

To conclude I would like to quote two references which help to illustrate the qualities to be encouraged in the general practitioner and which I think will be reflected in his consultations. The first was from an address by Will Pickles to medical students at Birmingham. At the end of his speech he said:

> 'I hope I have not been preaching, but I am going to finish up with something you may think of this nature. Never use the word "case", and never think the word "case". All those who come to you for treatment are individuals and often very frightened individuals and must receive the respect and consideration which one man owes another.'

The other is taken from a clinical/pathological conference, which was written up in the *British Medical Journal* in 1968 and was so well described by Dr Cerney (pseudonym) in Jonathan Gathorne-Hardy's book *Doctors*, that I have quoted it in full.

'It was a patient, just "A Man", and he had a terrible disease of his guts and all these clever doctors, professors of this and that and the other, took him to pieces, literally. They examined single enzyme systems in the lining of his gut. They almost took molecules of the poor man, and they got nowhere near finding out what was wrong with him. And after about fifteen years he died. And at the post-mortem conference when they looked at all the material, and all the medical contributors came, they also had his family doctor there and halfway through the Professor of Medicine turned to the family doctor and said, "Dr Hatfield, can you tell us something about the home life of this patient, as you may feel it has a bearing on it?" And the doctor said, "Yes, I think this man's illness started when his father died. Then it got much worse when his adopted daughter made what he regarded as an unsatisfactory marriage, and the final relapse, followed by his death, occurred when he was sacked from his job into which he'd put many, many years of hard work, and he was sacked without having any kind of adequate recompense made to him." And the Professor of Medicine said, "Yes, thank you very much, but I don't think really we can take psychological facts into account here. Professor Somebody, could you tell us about the something or other?" And they took absolutely no notice of that man, because doctors don't have a framework of reference to enable them to translate things like anger or sadness into diseases.'

Bibliography

Recently there has been considerable criticism levelled against trainee GPs for their lack of enthusiasm in reading medical literature. To help counteract this apparent apathy and encourage further reading. I have included in this bibliography a few additional comments and personal views about some of the books and articles mentioned.

Abercrombie, M. L. J. (1972). Non-verbal communication. *Proc. R. Soc. Med.*; **65:** 335–64.

Aitken-Swan, J., Easson, E. C. (1959). Reaction of cancer patients on being told their diagnosis. *Br. Med. J.;* **1:** 779–83.

Alexander, F., French, T. M., Bacon, C. L. *et al.* (1946). *Psychoanalytic Therapy: Principles and Application.* 1946, 1974, New York: John Wiley & Sons; 1980, Bison Book, Lincoln and London: University of Nebraska Press. *An introduction to the basic principles and application of psychoanalysis. Several authors, some more easy to read than others. Generally rewarding to read.*

Anderson, J. L. (1979). Patients' recall of information and its relation to the nature of the consultation. In *Research in Psychotherapy and Medicine* (Osborne *et al.*, eds.). London: Academic Press.

Apley, V. (1980). Communicating with children. *Br. Med. J.;* **281:** 1116–17.

Asher, R. (1955). Talk, tact and treatment. *Lancet*; **1:** 758–60.

Bain, D. J. (1976) Doctor–patient communication in general practice consultations. *Med. Educ.;* **10** (2); 125–131.

Bain, D. J. (1977). Patient knowledge and the content of the consultation in general practice. *Med. Educ.;* **11:** 347–50.

Balint, M. (1964). *The Doctor, his Patient and the Illness.* London: Pitman Medical. *First published in 1957, a preview of it was written by Balint in 1955 in* The Lancet; **268:** 681. *Widely acclaimed. Probably more than any other doctor in the last thirty years, Balint has influenced the course of general practice. Perhaps because English was not his native language, this book is not easy to read. Trainees should not be discouraged by this. There is so much to digest that it may be read several times to the reader's advantage.*

Balint, E., Norell, J. S., eds. (1973). *Six Minutes for the Patient: Interactions in General Practice Consultation.* London: Tavistock Publications. *Interesting but less convincing and less influential than Michael Balint's book. Good chapter by Cyril Gill.*

Barber, H. (1948). The act of dying. *Practitioner*; **161:** 76–79.

Barrows, H. S., Flightner, J. W., Neufield, V. R. *et al.* (1978). *An Analysis of the Clinical Methods of Medical Students and Physicians.* Hamilton, Ontario: McMaster University.

Baur, S. (1988). *Hypochondria: Woeful Imaginings.* Berkeley: University of California Press.

Becker, M. H. (1979). Understanding patient compliance: the contributions of attitudes and the psychological factors. In *New Directions in Patient Compliance*, (Cohen, S. J., ed.). Lexington, Mass.: Lexington Books.

Becker, M. H., Maiman, L. A. (1975). Sociobehavioural determinants of compliance with health and medical care recommendations. *Med. Care*; **13**: 10–14.

Bennett, A. E., ed. (1976). *Communication Between Doctors and Patients*, Contributors: Fraser, C., Johnston, M., Maguire, P., Rutter, D., Ley, P., Fishbein, M. Published for the Nuffield Provincial Hospitals Trust (London) by Oxford University Press (Oxford).

Bennett, A., Knox, J. D. E., Morrison, A. T. (1978). Difficulties in consultations reported by doctors in general practice. *J. R. Coll. Gen. Pract.*; **28**: 646–51.

Bennett, A., Morrison, A. J., Knox, J. D. (1979). Common sense and consulting. *J. R. Coll. Gen. Prac.*; **29** (201): 209–15.

Bennett, G. (1979). *Patients and their Doctors*. London: Baillière Tindall.

Berger, J. (1969). *A Fortunate Man*. London: Writers and Readers Publishing Cooperative Society.
An excellent study of a rural GP in the Forest of Dean. Beautifully written by the art critic, John Berger, it paints the best description I have yet read of 'character unfolding' in a GP.

Berne, E. (1973). *The Games People Play*. Harmondsworth, Middlesex: Penguin.
A somewhat idiosyncratic account of the ways in which people react to each other. His description of the games people play with one another may seem too schematic, unconvincing and even, possibly, irritating.

Bertakis, K. D. (1977). The communication of information from physician to patient: a method for increasing patient retention and satisfaction. *J. Fam. Pract.*; **5** (2); 217–22.

Bird, B. (1955). *Talking with Patients*. Philadelphia and Montreal: J. B. Lippincott.

Bloom, A. (1985) (Chairman of the Executive Council of the British Diabetic Association). Personal communication.

Bloom, S. W. (1963). *The Doctor and his Patient*. New York: Russell Sage Foundation.

Boranic, M. (1979). Silent information. *J. Med. Ethics*; **5** (2): 80–2.

Boyle, C. M. (1970). Differences between patients' and doctors' interpretations of some common medical terms. *Br. Med. J.*; **2**: 286–9.

Bräutigan, W., Knauss, W., Wolff, H. H. (1985). *First Steps in Psychotherapy*. Contributions from: Becker, H., Bloomfield, I., Bräutigam, W., Knauss, W., Senf, W., Sturgeon, D. and Wolff, H. H. Berlin, Heidelberg, New York, Tokyo: Springer Verlag.
A book for medical students and GPs. It is written in two parts; the first aims to improve the doctor's understanding of psychological mechanisms; the second describes the therapeutic mechanisms used in a typical Balint Group.

Brewin, T. B. (1977). The cancer patient: communication and morale. *Br. Med. J.*; **3**: 1623–7.
Well-written article on talking and listening to patients who are dying. Good description of the different phases of patients' reactions.

British Medical Association Planning Unit Report No. 4 (1970). *Report of the Working Party on Primary Medical Care*. London: BMA.

British Medical Journal (1963). Hospital manners. *Br. Med. J.*; **2**: 265–6.

Brooke, B. N. (1960). Broadening the clinical approach. *Lancet*; **2**: 810–12.

Brown, E. W., Harris, T. (1978). *Special Origins of Depression*. London: Tavistock Publications.

Browne, K., Freeling, P. (1967). *The Doctor-Patient Relationship*. Edinburgh & London: Churchill Livingstone.
Originally printed as a series of articles in The Practitioner in 1966; Compiled as a book and illustrated by case histories. Now in its third edition—Freeling, P. and Harris, C. Strongly recommended reading for all trainees.

Browne, K., Freeling, P. (1985). A basic misunderstanding. *Lancet*; **1**: 803–5.

Butler, J. R. (1980). *How Many Patients*. A study of list sizes in general practice. London: Bedford Square Press of the National Council for Voluntary Organisations.

Byrne, P. S. (1976). Teaching and learning verbal behaviours. In *Language and Communication in General Practice*. (Tanner, B., ed.) pp 52–70. London: Hodder & Stoughton.

Byrne, P. S., Long, B. E. L. (1976). *Doctors Talking to Patients*. A study of the verbal behaviour of general practitioners consulting in their surgery. London: HMSO, republished 1984: Royal College of General Practitioners.
A collection and analysis of hundreds of transcribed GP consultations. An excellent and entertaining book which, being out of print, was rightly published by the RCGP.

Calnan, J. (1983). *Talking with Patients—a Guide to Good Practice*. London: William Heinemann Medical Books.
Guide for medical students and hospital-based doctors to help improve their consultation and medical practice. Suffers from being rather didactic; reads like a catechism.

Carstairs, G. M. (1963). *This Island Now*. London: Hogarth Press.

Carstairs, V. (1970). *Channels of Communication*. Report on an enquiry carried out in Scotland for the Working Party on Suggestions and Complaints in Hospitals. Scottish Health Service Studies No. 11, Scottish Home and Health Department.

Cartwright, A. (1964). *Human Relations and Hospital Care*. London: Routledge and Kegan Paul.

Cartwright, A. (1967). *Patients and their Doctors. A Study of General Practice*. London: Routledge and Kegan Paul.

Cartwright, A., Anderson, R. (1981). *General Practice Revisited. A Second Study of Patients and their Doctors*. London: Tavistock Publications.
These three sociological surveys by Ann Cartwright were compiled over seventeen years. They reveal the alarming shortcomings of general practice, and particularly the failure of GPs to modify their consultation techniques to suit the obvious needs of the public.

Central Health Services Council (1963). *Communication between Doctors, Nurses and Patients. An Aspect of Human Relations in the Hospital Service*. London: HMSO.

Cohen, G. L. (1964). *What's Wrong with Hospitals?* London: Penguin Books.

Cole, B. S. (1982). Teaching medical interviewing in vocational training. *J. R. Coll. Gen. Pract.*; **32**: 665–72.

Committee on Hospital Complaints Procedure (1973). *Report* (Davies Report). London: HMSO.

Congalton, A. A. (1969). Public evaluation of medical care. *Med. J. Aust.*; **2:** 1165.

Cooke, A. (1986). *The Patient has the Floor*. London: The Bodley Head.
A series of addresses mainly to medical meetings. Witty, scholarly and humorous. Well crafted and moves with the rhythm of the spoken voice.

Coope, J., Metcalfe, D. (1979). How much do patients know? *J. R. Coll. Gen. Pract.* **29:** 482–8.

Cramond, W. A. (1970). Psychotherapy of the dying patient. *Br. Med. J.*; **3:** 389–93.

Earll, L., Kincey, J. (1982). Clinical psychology in general practice: a controlled trial evaluation. *J. R. Coll. Gen. Pract.*; **32:** 32–37.

Eastman, C., McPherson, I. (1982). As others see us. General practitioners' perceptions of psychological problems and the relevance of clinical psychology. *Br. J. Clin. Psychol.*; **21:** 85–92.

Ekman, P., Friesen, W. V., Ellsworth, P. (1972). *Emotion in the Human Face: Guidelines for Research and an Integration of Findings*. Pergamon Press: New York.

Elder, A., Samuel, O. (1987). 'While I'm here, doctor': a study of the doctor patient relationship. London: Tavistock Publications.

Ellenberger, H. (1970). *The Discovery of the Unconscious*. London: Allen Lane, The Penguin Press.

Elstein, A. S., Schulman, L. S., Sprafha, S. A. (1978). *Medical Problem Solving: an Analysis of Clinical Reasoning*. Cambridge, Mass.: Harvard University Press.

Engel, G. L. (1971). The deficiences of the case presentation as a method of clinical teaching. *New Eng. J. Med.*; **284:** 20–4.

Ferguson, L. K., Kerr, J. H. (1971). *Explain it to Me Doctor*. Philadelphia and Toronto: J. B. Lippincott.

Field, S., Jeffrey, D., Wright, P. (1995). The use of Drama to improve communication and consultation skills of trainee general practitioners. *Education for General Practice*; **6:** 214–17.

Fink, D. L. (1976). Tailoring the consensual regimen. In *Compliance with Therapeutic Regimens* (Sackett, D. L., Haynes, R. B., eds.). Baltimore: Johns Hopkins University Press.

Fitton, F., Acheson, H. W. K. (1979). *The Doctor–Patient Relationship. A Study in General Practice*. London: HMSO.
Well-written and well-researched study of the GP–patient relationship. Incorporates extensive sociological research. Highly recommended reading.

Fletcher, C. M. (1972). *Communication in Medicine*. The Rock Carling Fellowship. Nuffield Provincial Hospitals Trust.
Excellent first chapter on communicating and patients. Extensive bibliography.

Fletcher, C. M. (1980). Listening and talking to patients. *Br. Med. J.*; **281:** 845–7, 931–3, 994–6, 1056–8.
Series of articles, simply written and clearly expressed with great sensitivity. Easy to read.

Fox, T. F. (1962). Personal Medicine. *Bull. N. Y. Acad. Med.*; **38:** 527.

Francis, V., Korsch, B. M., Morris, M. J. (1969). Gaps in doctor–patient communication. Patients' response to medical advice. *New Eng. J. Med.*; **280:** 535–40.

Fraser, C. (1976). Analysis of face to face communication. In *Communication between Doctors and Patients* (Bennett, A. E., ed.), Nuffield Provincial Hospitals Trust; Oxford University Press.

Freeman, J., Byrne, P. S. (1976). *The Assessment of Vocational Training for General Practice*. Report from General Practice No. 17. London: Council of the Royal College of General Practitioners.

Freidson, E. (1962). Dilemmas in the doctor–patient relationship. In *Human Behaviour and Social Processes*, (Rose, A. M., ed.) Chapter 11. London: Routlege and Kegan Paul.

Friel, P. B. (1982). Death and dying. *Ann. Intern. Med.*; **97:** 767–71.
Clear and well-written account of the psychological processes involved in dying.

Froehlich, R. E. (1969). A course in medical interviewing. *J. Med. Educ.*; **44:** 1165.

Fry, J. (1983). *Common Dilemmas in Family Medicine*. Lancaster: MTP Press.
Medical moot topics argued by different authors.

Fry, J. (1983). *Present State and Future Needs in General Practice*, 6th edn. Lancaster: MTP Press. Published for the Royal College of General Practitioners.
Simple and well-presented book about the changes which will have to be incorporated into general practice in order to accommodate the future needs of the nation.

Gardner, K. (1985). Let your patients help. (Pulse Patient Leaflets Award Winner) *Pulse*; **45** (21): 41–48.

Gathorne-Hardy, J. (1984). *Doctors*. London: Weidenfeld & Nicholson.
Collection of interviews by Gathorne-Hardy with a great many GPs around the country. Very well compiled. Full of oblique references; parts of it rather depressing. Fascinating reading.

Gill, C. (1972). Types of interview in general practice. In *Patient Centred Medicine*, (Hopkins, P., ed.). London: Regional Doctor Publications.
Well-written chapter in a book that some might consider heavy going.

Golden, J. S., Johnston, C. D. (1970). Problems of distortion in doctor–patient communications. *Psychiatr. Med.*; **1:** 127–49.

Hampton, J. R., Harrison, M. J. E., Mitchell, J. R. A., Pritchard, J. S., Seymour, C. (1975). Relative contributions of history taking, physical examination and laboratory investigation to diagnosis and management of medical outpatients. *Br. Med. J.*; **2:** 486–9.

Hannay, D. R. (1979). *The Symptom Iceberg*. London: Routledge and Kegan Paul.

Hannay, D. R. (1980). The 'iceberg' of illness and 'trivial' consultations. *J. R. Coll. Gen. Pract.*; **30:** 551–4.
Two interesting accounts of the different perceptions of symptoms between doctors and patients. A comparison of those symptoms which are regarded as trivial and those which reveal serious underlying illness.

Hawkins, C. F. (1967). *Speaking and Writing in Medicine*. Springfield, Illinois: Charles C. Thomas.

Hawkins, C. F. (1968). Personal view. *Br. Med. J.*; **4:** 640.

Hawkins, C. (1979). Patients' reactions to their investigations: a study of 504 patients. *Br. Med. J.*; **2:** 638–40.

Hayes, D. M., Hutaff, L. W., Mace, D. R. (1971). Preparation of medical students for patient interviewing. *J. Med. Educ.*; **46:** 863–8.

Helfer, R. E. (1970). An objective comparison of the pediatric interviewing skills of freshmen and senior medical students. *Pediatrics*; **45**: 623–7.

Helman, C. G. (1981). Diseases versus illness in general practice. *J. R. Coll. Gen. Pract.*; **31**: 548–52.

Hinton, J. M. (1963). The physical and mental distress of the dying. *Q. J. Med.*; **32**: 1–21.

Honigsbaum, F. (1979). *The Division in British Medicine*. London: Kogan Page.

Hopkins, P., ed. (1972). *Patient-centred Medicine*. London: Regional Doctor Publications Ltd.

Horder, T. (1948). Signs and symptoms of impending death. *Practitioner*, **161**: 73–75.

Houghton, H. (1968). Problems of hospital communication: an experimental study. In '*Problems and Progress in Medical Care*', 3rd Series, (McLachlan, G., ed.). Oxford University Press for the Nuffield Provincial Hospitals Trust.

Howie, J. (1984). General practice: choice before change. *Mod. Med.*; May: 10–13.

Hugh-Jones, P., Tauser, A. R., Whitby, C. (1964). Patients' views of admission to a London teaching hospital. *Br. Med. J.*; **2**: 660–4.

Illich, I. (1975). *Medical Nemesis*. London: Calder & Boyars.

Illich, I. (1977). *Limits to Medicine*. Harmondsworth: Penguin Books Ltd.

Jason, H., Kagan, N., Werner, A., Elstein, A. S., Thomas, J. B. (1971). New approaches to teaching basic interview skills to medical students. *Am. J. Psychiat.*; **127**: 1404–7.

Jefferys, M., Sachs, H. (1983). *Rethinking General Practice. Dilemmas in Primary Medical Care*. London and New York: Tavistock Publications.

Klein, R. (1973). *Complaints Against Doctors*. London: Charles Knight.

Kleinman, A. (1980). *Patients and Healers in the Context of Culture*. Berkeley: University of California Press.

Knox, J. D. E., Alexander, D. W., Morrison, A. T. *et al.* (1979). Communication skills and undergraduate medical education. *Med. Educ.*, **13**: 345–8.

An analysis of medical consultations recorded on videotape. A brief but interesting comparison of consultations by medical students with those by postgraduate trainee GPs.

Korsch, B. M., Gozzi, E. K., Francis, V. (1968). Gaps in doctor–patient communication. 1. Doctor–patient interaction and patient satisfaction. *Pediatrics*; **42**: 855–71.

Krantz, D. S., Baum, A., Wideman, M. (1980). Assessment of preferences for self-treatment and information in health care. *J. Pers. Soc. Psychol.*; **39**: 977–90.

Lader, M. (1981). Benzodiazepine dependence. In *The Misuse of Psychotropic Drugs* (Murray, R. *et al.*, eds.). London: Gaskell Special Publications No. 1.

Laing, R. D. (1959). *The Divided Self: an 'Existential Study in Sanity and Manners*. London: Tavistock Publication Ltd.

Larsen, K. M., Smith, C. K. (1981). Assessment of non-verbal communication in the patient-physician interview. *J. Fam. Pract.*; **12**: 481–8.

Ley, P. (1976). Towards better doctor–patient communications. In *Communications Between Doctors and Patients*, (Bennett, A. E., ed.). London: OUP for Nuffield Provincial Hospitals Trust.

Ley, P., Spelman, M. S. (1967). *Communicating with the Patient.* London: Staple Press.
Survey of what patients know, and how well they recall information passed on to them during the consultation: how this relates to compliance, and how misunderstanding and confusion arise.

Ley, P., Whitworth, M., Skilbeck, C. *et al.* (1976). Improving doctor–patient communications in general practice. *J. R. Coll. Gen. Pract.,* **26:** 720–4.

Livesey, P. G. (1986). *Partners in Care: The Consultation in General Practice.* London: Heinemann Medical.

Lochman, J. E., Dain, R. N., Fogleman, J. D., Sullivan, D. H. (1981). Interviewing skills training in a family practice residency program. *J. Fam. Pract.;* **12:** 1080–1.

Long, B. E. L. (1974). Doctors talking to patients: verbal communication. *Gen. Prac. Inter.;* **4:** 152–8.

Long, B. (1984). Patient watching. *Pulse;* March 10, p. 25.

McGhee, A. (1961). *The Patient's Attitude to Nursing Care.* Edinburgh and London: E. & S. Livingstone.

MacKenzie, J. (1916). *The Principles of Diagnosis and Treatment in Heart Afflictions.* London: Hodder & Stoughton.

Macleod, J. ed. (1964). *Clinical Examination.* 2nd edn. London: Churchill.

McWhinney, I. R. (1981). *An Introduction to Family Medicine.* Oxford: Oxford University Press.

Maguire, G. P., Rutter, D. R. (1976). History-taking for medical students. 1. Deficiences in performance. *Lancet,* **2:** 556–8.

Maguire, G. P., Rutter, D. R. (1976). Training medical students to communicate—development of an interviewing model. In *Communication Between Doctors and Patients* (Bennett, A. E., ed.). Oxford: Nuffield Provincial Hospitals Trust and Oxford University Press.
Clearly written chapter about communication between patients and doctors. Discussion about medical students and their common faults with interview technique.

Marinker, M. (1972). *Repeat Prescriptions In Patient-centred Medicine,* (Hopkins, P., ed.). London: Regional Doctor Publications Ltd.

Marinker, M. (1984). *A New NHS Act for 1996?* London: OHE.

Marks, J. N., Goldberg, D. P., Hillier, V. F. (1979). Determinants of the ability of general practitioners to detect psychiatric illness. *Psychol. Med.;* **9:** 337–53.

Martin, P. (1983). Receptionists—a GP's guide to their selection and training. *Pulse:* 15 October, 31–8.
Useful guide to the selection of receptionists, the importance of which has been much underrated.

Massarik, F., Wechsler, I. R. (1959). Empathy Revisited: The Process of Understanding People. *California Management Review* Vol. 1 No. 2, 36–46. From: Kolb, D. A., Rubin, I. M., McIntyre, J. M. (eds.) Organizational Psychology: Readings on Human Behaviour in Organizations. 4th edn Chapter 10 Interpersonal Perception. Prentice-Hall, New Jersey, USA.

Meares, A. (1960). Communication with the patient. *Lancet,* **1:** 663–7.

Mechanic, D. (1968). *Medical Sociology.* New York: Free Press.

Medaway, C. (1984). *The Wrong Kind of Medicine.* Hertford: Consumers Association publication.

Well-written account encouraging doctors to allow their patients greater participation in decisions. He maintains that a questioning patient is a vitally important safeguard to prescribing.

Medical Defence Union (1972). *Annual Report*, p. 33. London: Medical Defence Union.

Melville, J. (1985). *The Tranquillizer Trap and How to Get Out of It.* London: Fontana.
Harsh criticism of the medical profession. There is more than a grain of truth in her claims that GPs regarded tranquillizers as an answer to their own problems as much as to those of their patients.

Mendel, D. (1984). *Proper Doctoring.* Berlin: Springer Verlag.
Clearly-written book for hospital doctors. Didactic approach with an amusing idiosyncratic style.

Metcalfe, D. H. H., Hillier, S., Pritchard, P. M. M. *et al.* (1981). In *Patient Participation in General Practice* (Pritchard, P. M. M., ed.). London: Royal College of General Practitioners Occasional Paper 17.

Meyer, B. C. (1969). Truth and the physician. *Bull. N.Y. Acad. Med.*; **45:** 59–71.

Milligan, S. (1983). *Indefinite Articles and Scunthorpe.* London: Sphere.
Contains a disturbing account of the death of his wife. He argues that cancer victims should not be told the diagnosis.

Morris, D. (1977). *Manwatching. A field guide to human behaviour.* London: Jonathan Cape.

Neighbour, R. (1987). *The Inner Consultation.* Lancaster: Kluwer Academic.
Well-written account of the consultation. A unique view of how to improve the quality of the consultation by focusing attention on the functions of both our cerebral hemispheres: the left, the Organizer and the right, the Responder. Includes an excellent precis of the various consultation models. The text is slightly marred by curious typographical errors. Otherwise a marvellous book, now a classic. Should be essential reading.

Neighbour, R. (1992). *The Inner Apprentice.* Lancaster: Kluwer Academic.
Discusses the gap between potential and achievement with respect to GP Registrars. The 'Inner Apprentice' is our unconscious self-educating mechanism. We are all unsettled by our ignorance. This 'cognitive dissonance' may be usefully provoked and mobilized to improve learning.

O'Donnell, M. (1986). *Doctor! Doctor!: An Insider's Guide to the Games Doctors Play.* London: Victor Gollancz.
An amusing yet very pointed comment about general practice. Well written, it describes in detail what patients need in a doctor. It covers a wide range of topics and is a really enjoyable read. He also pokes fun at would-be academics with studied 'gravitas'.

Parish, P. (1971). The prescribing of psychotropic drugs. *J. R. Coll. Gen. Pract.*; **21:** Suppl 4, 61.

Parkes, C. M. (1973). Panel discussion: the patient's right to know the truth. Library and Lay Section. *Proc. E. Soc. Med.*; **66:** 533.

Parry, R. (1983). *Basic Psychotherapy.* Edinburgh: Churchill Livingstone.
Easy, simple introduction to psychotherapy.

Pemberton, J. (1970). *Will Pickles of Wensleydale: Life of a Country Doctor.* London: Geoffrey Bles.
Biography of Dr William Pickles, who practised in Aysgarth in the Yorkshire Dales. Easy and light-hearted, but trainees could learn a great deal from the attitudes that prevail throughout this book.

Pendleton, D., Hasler, J. eds. (1983). *Doctor-Patient Communication*. London: Academic Press: Harcourt Brace Jovanovich Publishers.

Pendleton, D., Schofield, T., Tate, P., Havelock, P. (1984). *The Consultation: an Approach to Learning and Teaching*. Oxford: Oxford Medical Publications.
  Really two books in one. The first half is a sociological view, advocating GPs to explore their patients' ideas and concerns. It is well argued and well written, and aimed at all GPs but especially trainees. The latter half is written for trainers and aims to help them assess and teach their trainees. It suffers from too much jargon and the advocated method of assessment seems cumbersome and could in some instances be inappropriate. Has become a classic text.

Pickles, W. N. (1939). *Epidemiology in Country Practice* (with preface by Professor Major Greenwood). Bristol: John Wright.
  A classical work of epidemiology, containing, among many things, a very good clinical description of Bornholm's disease.

Pietroni, P. (1976). Non-verbal communication in the general practice surgery. In *Language and Communication in General Practice*, (Tanner, B., ed.). London: Hodder & Stoughton.

Preece, J. (1994). *The Use of Computers in General Practice*. 3rd edn. London: Churchill Medical Communications.

Qureshi, B. (1989). *Transcultural Medicine: Dealing with Patients from Different Cultures*. Dordrecht: Kluwer Academic.

Raphael, W. (1969). *Patients and their Hospitals*. London: King Edward's Hospital Fund.

Raphael, W., Peers, V. (1972). *Psychiatric Hospitals Viewed by their Patients*. London: King Edward's Hospital Fund.

Raynes, N. V. (1980). A preliminary study of search procedures and patient management techniques in general practice. *J. R. Coll. Gen. Pract.*; **13:** 166–72.

Raynes, N. V., Cairns, V. (1980). Factors contributing to the length of general practice consultations. *J. R. Coll. Gen. Pract.*; **30:** 496–8.

Redlich, F. C. (1949). The patients' language. *Yale J. Biol. Med.*; **17:** 427–53.

Rees, W. D. (1972). The distress of dying. *Br. Med. J.*; **3:** 105–7.

Reynolds, M. (1978). No news is bad news: patients' views about communication in hospital. *Br. Med. J.*; **1:** 1673–6.

Rosenheim, Professor Lord (1972) Foreword to *Patient-centred Medicine* (Hopkins, P., ed.). London: Regional Doctor Publications Ltd.

Rosenstock, I. M. (1966). Why people use health services. *Millbank Mem. Fund Q.*; **44:** 94–127.

Royal College of General Practitioners (1972). *The Future General Practitioner—Learning and Teaching*. London: RCGP.

Samson-Fisher, R., Maguire, P. (1980). Should skills in communicating with patients be taught in medical schools? *Lancet*; **2:** 523–6.
  Good article advocating the training of medical students in better communication.

Saunders, C. (1959). Care of the dying. Reprinted from *Nursing Times*; **55:** 9, 16, 23, 30, October 6 and November 13.
  Articles on the now classical work of Dame Cicely Saunders.

Seligmann, A. W., McGrath, N. E., Pratt, L. (1957). Level of medical information among clinical patients. *J. Chronic. Dis.*; **6:** 497–509.

Bibliography · 131

Sheldon, M., Stoddart, N. (1985). *Trends in General Practice Computing.* London: RCGP.

Short, P. W. (1980). Why not discard the desk? *J. R. Coll. Gen. Pract.*; **30**: 687.

Brief article about the barrier to communication imposed by the relative position of the desk in relationship to the positions of doctor and patient.

Skipper, J. K. (1965). Communication and the hospitalized patient. In *Social Interaction and Patient Care*, (Skipper, J. K., Leonard, R. C., eds). Philadelphia: J. B. Lippincott.

Skipper, J. K., Tagliacozzo, D. L, Mauksh, H. O. (1964). Some possible consequences of limited communication between patients and hospital functionaries. *J. Health Human Behav.*; **5**: 34–39.

Skynner, R., Cleese, J. (1983). *Families and How to Survive Them.* London: Methuen.

Comedian and actor John Cleese, by chance, met his psychoanalyst Robin Skynner some while after analysis had been concluded. From this encounter evolved this book which reads as a transcription of a series of conversations between them. The theme is about the way members of a family react with one another. The style is idiosyncratic and light-hearted. Despite this however, the book has a serious purpose and one which could be helpful to trainees. Now available on audiocassette.

Spelman, M. S., Ley, P., Jones, C. (1966). How do we improve doctor-patient communication in our hospitals? *World Hospitals*; **2**: 126–9.

Spence, J. (1960). The need for understanding the individual as part of the training of doctors and nurses. In *The Purpose and Practice of Medicine.* London: Oxford University Press.

From this selection of writings by Sir James Spence Chapter XVIII is particularly relevant to doctors starting upon their career. Spence was Professor of Childhealth at Newcastle and a great friend of Will Pickles. He had a great respect for general practice.

Steward, M. A., McWhinney, I. R., Buck, C. W. (1979). The doctor–patient relationship and its effect upon outcome. *J. R. Coll. Gen. Pract.*; **29**: 77–82.

Stimson, G., Webb, B. (1975). *Going to See the Doctor. The Consultation Process in General Practice.* London and Boston: Routledge and Kegan Paul.

A comprehensive view of the consultation in general practice. Invaluable reading for the trainee GP.

Stott, N. C. H., Davis, R. H. (1979) The exceptional potential in each primary care consultation. *J. R. Coll. Gen. Pract.*; **29**: 201–5.

Stott, P. (1983). *Milestones, the Diary of a Trainee GP.* London and Sydney: Pan.

Interesting diary of a trainee GP. Well presented, with emphasis upon the psychological aspects of general practice.

Strauss, A., Schatzman, L., Bucher, R., Ehrlich, D., Sabshin, M. (1964). *Psychiatric Ideologies and Institutions.* London: Collier-Macmillan.

Strube, G. (1984). Leaflets reinforce advice from GPs to their patients. *Pulse*; January 14, 68.

Tähkä, V. (1984). *The Patient Doctor Relationship.* Sydney: Adis Health Science Press.

Regrettably this is not an easy book to read, possibly because of the difficulties with translation. However, despite this it is excellent, and should be better known than it is.

Tanner, B. A. ed. (1976). *Language and Communication in General Practice.* London: Hodder and Stoughton.

Tapia, F. (1972). Teaching medical interviewing: a practical technique. *Br. J. Med. Educ.*; **6**: 133–6.

Taylor, Lord (1954). *Good General Practice*. OUP/Nuffield Provincial Hospitals Trust.

Truax, C. B., Carkhuff, R. R. (1967). *Toward Effective Counselling and Psychotherapy: Training and Practice*. Chicago: Aldine.

Truax, C. B., Mitchell, K. M. (1971). *Handbook of Psychotherapy and Behavioural Change*, (Bergin, A. E., Garfield, S. L. eds). New York: Wiley.

Tuckett, D. ed. (1976). *An Introduction to Medical Sociology*. Tavistock Publications: London.

Tuckett, D. (1982). *Final Report on the Patient Project*. London: Health Education Council.
For some time, Tuckett has been encouraging GPs to explore their patient's ideas and concerns about their illnesses. D. Pendleton has recently popularized this idea.

Verby, J. E., Holden, P., Davis, R. M. (1979). Peer review of consultations in primary care: the use of audio-visual recordings. *Br. Med. J.*; **1**: 1686–8.

Waitzkin, H., Stoeckle, J. D. (1972). The communication of information about illness: clinical, social and methodological considerations. *Adv. Psychosom. Med.*; **8**: 180–215.

Walton, J., Duncan, A. S., Fletcher, C. M. *et al.* (1982). *Talking with Patients: a Teaching Approach*. Observations of a Nuffield Working Party on communications with patients. London: Nuffield Provincial Hospitals Trust.
Simple booklet with well-annotated bibliography by C. M. Fletcher.

Ward, N. G., Stein, L. (1975). Reducing emotional distance. A new method to teach interviewing skills. *J. Med. Educ.*; **50**: 605–14.

Waters, A., Macintyre, I. M. A. (1976). Attitudes and criticism of surgical in-patients. *Practitioner*, **218**: 269.

Watts, C. A. H. (1966). *Depressive Disorders in the Community*. Bristol: John Wright.
The realization that many problems in general practice could not be explained in terms of hospital medicine provided Watts with the stimulus to write this book, which has a more appropriate approach to depressive disorders in the community.

Watts, C. A. H. (1971). The hot line. *Br. Med. J.*; **3**: 419–21.

Wells, G. (1978). *How to Communicate*. London: McGraw-Hill.

White, L. P. (ed.) (1969). Conference on care of patients with fatal illness. *Ann. N. Y. Acad. Sci.*; **164**: 637–896.

Wilkinson, A., Stratta, L., Dudley, P. (1974). *The Quality of Listening*. London: Methuen.

Wilson, G. M. (1972). Prescribing for patients leaving hospital. *Prescribers' J.*; **12**: 63–68.

Woodall, J. (1996). Self Awareness (personal communication).

Woods, M. M. (1979). Problems in doctor–patient communication: a survey of 100 anaesthetic patients. *Aust. Psychol.*; **14**: 227.

Wright, H. J., Macadam, D. B. (1979). *Clinical Thinking and Practice (Diagnosis and Decision in Patient Care)*. Edinburgh: Churchill Livingstone.
A lucid account which attempts to persuade medical students to reconsider their clinical approach to patients.

Zola, I. K. (1972). Studying the decision to see a doctor; review, critique, corrective. In *Psychological Aspects of Physical Illness*, (Lipowski, Z. J., ed.). *Advances in Psychosomatic Medicine*, Vol. 8. Basel: Karger.

Videotape References

Brief Encounters 605. The MSD Foundation, Tavistock House, Tavistock Square, London WC1H 9LG. Telephone 0171 387 6881.

Problems in Doctor/Patient Encounters—Learning from one another (1986). Royal Society of Medicine (Film and Television). Produced in association with the University of Liverpool.

UK Summative Assessment Package, A Guide for GP Trainers and *Calibration Video* (1995). British Postgraduate Medical Federation, South (West) Thames Region (copies provided courtesy of Glaxo Wellcome).

Surgery Dilemma – Menorrhagia and the demanding patient (1988). Video Horizons, vol. 1 no. 5.

Surgery Dilemma – Another demanding patient: appetite suppressants (1988). Video Horizons, vol. 1, no. 6.

Index